THE BODY ENGINEERING

The Most Advanced Machine Ever Created

DR. RAJESH BHOIR

notionpress.com

INDIA • SINGAPORE • MALAYSIA

ISBN
Paperback 979-8-90231-853-8
Hardcase 979-8-90540-883-0

Contents

Introduction

The Body Engineering

Dr. Rajesh Bhoir

The human body represents the most sophisticated, intelligent, and resilient biological system known to science. Contemporary advances in systems biology, neuroscience, epigenetics, molecular medicine, and integrative physiology increasingly confirm a reality long articulated by classical medical traditions such as Ayurveda: the human organism is not a random assembly of organs, but a unified, self-regulating, and continuously adaptive living system. Each cell operates with embedded intelligence, responding to internal and external signals while contributing to the stability of the whole. No human-designed machine, regardless of technological advancement, rivals the depth of coordination, adaptability, and autonomy demonstrated by the human body. Unlike machines that require external commands, the body operates through intrinsic awareness, real-time feedback loops, and decentralized decision-making across cellular, tissue, and systemic levels.

Modern engineering marvels—jet engines, supercomputers, robotic systems, and artificial intelligence—are designed for specific functions under controlled parameters. They require predefined inputs, constant monitoring, scheduled shutdowns, and external maintenance. Even the most advanced artificial intelligence systems remain dependent on externally provided data, energy, and repair. In contrast, the human body performs millions of interconnected tasks simultaneously and continuously, without interruption, from conception until death. It regulates temperature, circulation, respiration, digestion, detoxification, immunity, tissue repair, cognition, emotional processing, and consciousness itself, while dynamically adapting to variations in environment, nutrition, stress, injury, and aging. From an engineering standpoint, this level of integration, redundancy, and adaptability far exceeds the capabilities of any man-made system.

At the core of this biological excellence lies a complex network of ultra-sensitive sensors and control mechanisms. The nervous system provides rapid electrical communication, the endocrine system delivers precise chemical signaling, the immune system performs intelligent surveillance and repair, and cellular feedback pathways constantly monitor energy balance, oxygen availability, and metabolic integrity. These systems work in synchrony to preserve homeostasis under fluctuating conditions. Minor deviations in pH, glucose, temperature, pressure, or inflammatory load are detected and corrected instantly. The body achieves extraordinary efficiency, generating immense functional output from relatively modest nutritional input. Its regenerative ability—though finite—allows for wound healing, tissue renewal, immune memory, and functional recovery unmatched by any artificial construct. These attributes firmly establish the human body as the most advanced self-operating biological machine ever observed.

Despite this remarkable design, modern human behavior reveals a striking paradox. Machines of far lesser complexity and value are maintained with meticulous discipline, while the human body is often neglected, overloaded, and misused. Industrial systems follow strict preventive protocols, calibrated fueling standards, load management strategies, and early repair schedules. Engineers never wait for total breakdown before intervention, knowing that late-stage failure is costly and often irreversible. In contrast, human health is frequently addressed only after dysfunction becomes severe, chronic, or structurally damaging. The body is routinely subjected to incompatible nutrition, prolonged stress, disrupted sleep, sedentary habits, and environmental toxins, yet medical attention is often sought only when symptoms become disabling.

During my 11 years of medical practice, I have had the privilege of treating thousands of patients from diverse backgrounds, age groups, and lifestyles. One observation has remained remarkably consistent throughout this journey: the majority of people are unaware of the fundamental principles of preventive health care. Nearly 90–95% of patients I encounter lack adequate knowledge about proper nutrition, healthy lifestyle habits, disease prevention, and the maintenance of physical and mental well-being. Most individuals seek medical attention only after illness develops, rather than taking proactive steps to preserve their health. This book, The Body Engineering, is an effort to bridge that knowledge gap. Just as a complex machine requires regular maintenance, the human body also demands proper care, nourishment, and disciplined living to function at its best. Through this book, I aim to highlight common mistakes people make in their daily lives, explain the science behind healthy living in simple language, and provide practical guidance that can help individuals take control of their health before disease takes control of them.

The consequences of this neglect are evident worldwide. Chronic disorders such as diabetes, hypertension, cardiovascular disease, autoimmune conditions, degenerative joint disorders, infertility, metabolic syndrome, and neurodegenerative diseases have reached epidemic proportions. These conditions are commonly attributed to aging, genetics, or fate. However, both engineering logic and biological science demonstrate that complex systems do not fail suddenly. They deteriorate progressively through stages of imbalance, inefficiency, overload, inflammation, and micro-damage long before overt failure becomes apparent. The human body obeys the same universal principles that govern all complex systems.

Biological systems continuously generate early warning signals. Fatigue, stiffness, pain, digestive irregularities, sleep disturbances, emotional volatility, reduced endurance, and declining mental clarity are not random inconveniences. They are precise diagnostic messages indicating deviation from optimal function. In engineering terms, these are alarm signals designed to trigger timely correction. Unfortunately, contemporary healthcare culture often suppresses these signals through symptomatic treatment without addressing underlying causes. This approach is analogous to disabling warning alarms in a malfunctioning machine while allowing internal damage to progress unnoticed.

Ayurveda offered a profound understanding of this process thousands of years ago. It described disease as a gradual loss of functional harmony, unfolding through predictable stages before structural damage becomes evident. This insight aligns precisely with modern concepts of pathophysiology, systems failure, and disease progression. Correction at the functional stage—when imbalance is reversible—requires minimal intervention and yields durable outcomes. Once pathology becomes structural, manifesting as tissue destruction or organ dysfunction, restoration becomes complex, expensive, and often incomplete. Modern medicine demonstrates extraordinary excellence in managing advanced disease through surgery, pharmacology, critical care, and life-support technologies. Ayurveda complements this strength by emphasizing early detection, preventive maintenance, and restoration of regulatory balance.

Fuel quality represents another fundamental engineering principle with direct biological relevance. No high-performance engine can function efficiently on incompatible fuel. Even minor deviations in fuel composition gradually impair performance and shorten operational lifespan. Similarly, the human metabolic system depends on food that aligns with digestive capacity, biological rhythms, and individual constitution. Modern dietary patterns—dominated by ultra-processed foods, refined sugars, artificial additives, trans fats, and erratic eating schedules—overload metabolic pathways. Digestion becomes incomplete, metabolic waste accumulates, inflammation becomes chronic, and hormonal coordination deteriorates. Contemporary science recognizes these outcomes as insulin resistance, dysbiosis, metabolic syndrome, and chronic low-grade inflammation.

Ayurveda described the same phenomenon through the concept of *Ama*, referring to toxic, undigested metabolic byproducts that obstruct physiological pathways and initiate disease. From an engineering perspective, this represents contamination of the fuel processing system. Importantly, modern nutritional science, gastroenterology, and endocrinology increasingly validate this framework, demonstrating convergence rather than contradiction between ancient insight and contemporary evidence.

Equally damaging is chronic overload. All engineered systems are designed with defined load capacities and recovery requirements. Continuous operation beyond these limits accelerates wear and precipitates failure. The human nervous system evolved to manage acute stress followed by recovery. Modern life, however, imposes continuous cognitive, emotional, and sensory load without adequate rest. Persistent performance pressure, sleep deprivation, emotional suppression, and digital overstimulation keep stress pathways chronically activated. This disrupts neuroendocrine balance, suppresses immunity, impairs repair mechanisms, and accelerates degeneration.

As a result, psychological stress manifests as physical disease. Hypertension, gastrointestinal disorders, autoimmune conditions, infertility, depression, and cardiovascular disease emerge not as isolated disorders, but as systemic consequences of prolonged overload. Ayurveda recognized this interconnection by emphasizing the role of mental and emotional regulation in preserving physiological harmony. Modern neuroscience and psychoneuroimmunology now provide measurable evidence for this relationship, reinforcing the necessity of integrative approaches.

Modern healthcare systems excel in crisis intervention and advanced repair. Dialysis replaces renal function, joint replacement restores mobility, bypass surgery saves ischemic myocardium, and immunomodulatory drugs control life-threatening inflammation. These achievements represent the pinnacle of scientific and technological progress. However, they primarily address outcomes rather than origins. Ayurveda placed preventive maintenance at the core of medical responsibility, asserting that preserving the health of the healthy is the highest goal of medicine. Both perspectives are essential: one rescues life during failure, the other prevents failure from occurring.

The Body Engineering is founded on the understanding that health follows universal engineering laws. Health is not accidental, and disease is not inevitable. The human body is designed for longevity, resilience, and sustained performance when maintained in accordance with its biological blueprint. This work proposes a paradigm shift—from reactive treatment to preventive maintenance, from symptom suppression to system optimization, and from fragmented interventions to integrated biological engineering. By respectfully uniting the precision of modern medicine with the holistic intelligence of Ayurveda, this book offers a rational, sustainable, and scientifically grounded framework for lifelong health preservation.

Classical wisdom reminds us that the body is the primary instrument through which human potential is expressed. An instrument neglected cannot perform, a machine without maintenance cannot deliver output, and a body without engineering discipline cannot sustain health. Understanding the human body as an engineered system is not a philosophical abstraction; it is the foundation of a truly preventive, integrative, and future-ready model of medicine.

Purpose of This Book

The Body Engineering exists to restore engineering logic to human health. It does not oppose modern medicine—it completes it. Repair without prevention is incomplete. Prevention without science is inadequate. Integration is essential.

The greatest engineering error of modern civilization is assuming infinite repair capacity in biology. Neurons, nephrons, cartilage, and beta cells, once lost, are rarely restored.

When medicine and engineering think together, health stops being accidental—and becomes designed.

Chapter 1

The Human Body: The Most Advanced Engine Ever Created

Dr. Rajesh Bhoir

The human body stands as the most advanced engineering system ever known, not merely because of its astonishing complexity, but because of its intrinsic intelligence, adaptability, self-awareness, and self-preserving capacity. Modern science has built machines of extraordinary sophistication—jet engines capable of operating under immense thermal stress, nuclear reactors sustaining controlled energy release, supercomputers performing trillions of calculations per second, and artificial intelligence systems capable of learning, pattern recognition, and predictive analytics. Yet, despite their technological brilliance, all such systems remain fundamentally dependent on external design, external control, external maintenance, and external intelligence. The human body, in contrast, is a living system that designs, powers, regulates, repairs, optimizes, and sustains itself from within.

From an engineering perspective, this distinction is profound. No man-made machine can autonomously sense its own internal imbalance, predict its future failure, repair microscopic damage before breakdown, adapt its performance strategy based on the environment, and simultaneously generate subjective experience and consciousness. The human body does all of this continuously, silently, and efficiently for decades. It does not merely function—it *understands* its own functioning.

Ayurveda articulated this truth with remarkable clarity thousands of years ago:

> **"Yantra-vat śarīram"**
> *The human body functions like a perfectly designed machine*
> — *Charaka Samhita, Sharira Sthana*

This statement does not imply mechanical rigidity. Rather, it recognizes the body as the highest form of **living engineering**, far superior to inert machinery because it possesses awareness, adaptability, and regenerative intelligence. Unlike machines that fail abruptly when a single component malfunctions, the human body compensates, redistributes load, reroutes function, and delays failure—often for years—before breakdown becomes clinically visible.

1.1 The Body as a Living Engineering Network

The human body cannot be correctly understood by studying organs in isolation, just as a city cannot be understood by looking only at its buildings. The body functions as a living engineering network in which every system is connected, communicates continuously, and adjusts its behavior based on the condition of other systems. Electrical signals travel through nerves within milliseconds, chemical messengers such as hormones circulate through blood over minutes to hours, immune signals respond dynamically to threats, and mechanical forces generated by muscles, blood flow, and posture influence cellular behavior. Alongside these measurable pathways exist subtle bioenergetic and biochemical cues that fine-tune function at the cellular level. Because of this constant communication, no organ truly works alone. The brain influences the gut, the gut affects immunity, immunity alters metabolism, metabolism impacts hormones, and hormones shape mood and behavior. Health is the result of this synchronized communication, not the perfection of any single part.

To understand this in simple terms, the body can be compared to a self-governing city that never sleeps. Each cell is like a citizen with a specific job—some produce energy, some build structure, some defend against threats, and others manage information. Mitochondria act like power plants, generating energy needed for all activities. Roads and communication lines are represented by blood vessels, nerves, and lymphatic channels, ensuring rapid transport of materials and information. Hormones act like official letters or digital messages, coordinating long-term planning such as growth, reproduction, and stress adaptation. The liver, kidneys, lungs, intestines, and skin work like sanitation and waste-processing departments, constantly removing garbage so that the city remains clean and functional. Repair teams—stem cells, immune cells, and repair enzymes—operate silently in the background, fixing damage before it becomes visible. The brain and autonomic nervous system act as the central administration, continuously monitoring conditions and reallocating resources. During sleep, the city does not shut down; instead, it switches to maintenance mode—repairing tissues, clearing waste from the brain, reorganizing memory, and restoring energy reserves.

Modern systems biology strongly supports this integrated view of health. Research now shows that disturbances in one system inevitably affect others. For example, chronic stress originating in the mind alters hormonal signaling, which disrupts digestion, weakens immunity, raises blood sugar, and increases inflammation throughout the body. Similarly, poor gut health does not remain confined to digestion; it can influence mood, immunity, skin health, and even brain function through the gut-brain axis. A person with persistent indigestion, fatigue, and anxiety may have normal scans and reports for individual organs, yet the network as a whole is malfunctioning. This explains why treating only one organ often provides temporary relief but not lasting health.

Ayurveda recognized this network intelligence thousands of years ago by describing the body as a coordinated system governed by Dosha, Agni, Dhatu, Mala, and Manas. It emphasized that health arises when these elements remain in harmony. Disease, in this view, is not an external enemy suddenly attacking the body, but a gradual loss of coordination within the system. When communication breaks down—when digestion is weak, stress is excessive, waste is not eliminated properly, or daily rhythms are ignored—the network becomes inefficient. Over time, this inefficiency localizes in weaker areas, eventually appearing as disease. In simple language, disease is like traffic.

1.2 The Great Paradox of Modern Civilization

Despite the human body being the most advanced and irreplaceable engineering system ever created, modern civilization treats it with far less care than it gives to machines. This paradox lies at the heart of the global explosion of chronic disease. In every field of engineering, preventive care is considered common sense. Vehicles are serviced at fixed intervals, even when they appear to be running smoothly. Aircraft are grounded if even a small sensor shows abnormal readings, because engineers understand that minor faults, if ignored, can lead to catastrophic failure. Industrial machines are equipped with continuous monitoring systems that track vibration, temperature, pressure, and efficiency. Any deviation from optimal parameters triggers immediate inspection and correction. No responsible engineer waits for a complete breakdown before taking action.

In sharp contrast, the human body is routinely pushed far beyond its design limits. Sleep deprivation is accepted as a sign of ambition rather than as a warning of neurological and hormonal strain. Chronic stress is praised as dedication, even though it continuously overloads the nervous and endocrine systems. Food is chosen for convenience, taste, or marketing rather than biological compatibility, leading to metabolic overload and inflammation. Natural urges such as hunger, thirst, defecation, rest, and emotional expression are repeatedly suppressed in the name of productivity and social norms. Early warning signals—fatigue, indigestion, stiffness, disturbed sleep, mood changes—are dismissed as "normal" or managed with temporary relief measures instead of correction. Medical care is often sought only when damage has progressed to a stage where reversal is difficult or impossible.

A Simple example makes this Contradiction Clear. No one would drive a car for years without changing engine oil, coolant, or brake fluid and then be surprised when the engine seizes. Yet people routinely ignore the body's need for rest, nourishment, hydration, and recovery for decades and then express shock when diabetes, hypertension, joint degeneration, or heart disease appears. In engineering, such behavior would be labeled misuse or neglect. In human health, it is often mistaken for bad luck or unavoidable aging. This misunderstanding allows preventable diseases to flourish despite advances in diagnostics and treatment.

From an engineering standpoint, this approach is not just irrational—it is negligent. Chronic diseases dominate modern morbidity not because medicine has failed, but because the operating principles of the human body are routinely violated. Modern medicine excels at repair after failure—surgeries, drugs, intensive care, and life-support systems save lives and reduce suffering. However, no amount of advanced repair can fully compensate for years of incorrect operation. Ayurveda recognized this fundamental truth thousands of years ago and identified the root cause as **Pragyaparadha,** the failure of judgment or misuse of intelligence.

> **"Pragyāparādha eva sarva roganām mūlam"**
> *Failure of judgment is the root cause of all diseases*
>
> — *Charaka Samhita*

In simple terms, this means knowing what is harmful and still doing it, or knowing what is necessary and still ignoring it. In modern engineering language, this is best described as **operator error**. The machine is not faulty; the way it is used is. When the operator ignores warning signs, overloads the system, uses the wrong inputs, and delays maintenance, failure becomes inevitable. The same principle applies to the human body. Disease, in this light, is not betrayal by the body but the final outcome of long-standing misuse. Understanding this paradox shifts the focus of healthcare from blame and fear toward responsibility, awareness, and intelligent self-management—the foundation of true preventive medicine.

1.3 The Genetic Blueprint: Adaptive Design, Not Fixed Destiny

Every engineered system begins with a blueprint, a master plan that determines structure, function, limits, and repair capacity. In the human body, this blueprint is encoded in DNA, the most sophisticated design architecture ever discovered. The human genome consists of billions of precisely arranged base pairs that guide embryological development, organ formation, cellular specialization, metabolism, immunity, tissue repair, and even aging patterns. This blueprint is so comprehensive that a single fertilized cell, carrying microscopic strands of DNA, can eventually generate a complete human being with trillions of specialized cells working in harmony. From an engineering viewpoint, no design created by humans comes close to this level of informational density, efficiency, and foresight.

However, unlike mechanical blueprints—which are fixed, rigid, and unchanging—the biological blueprint is dynamic and responsive. Every cell in the body contains the complete genetic instruction manual, yet a brain cell behaves very differently from a liver cell or a muscle cell. This difference does not arise because the DNA is different, but because different sections of the same blueprint are activated or silenced according to function, location, and need. This process is controlled by epigenetic mechanisms—chemical tags and regulatory signals that turn genes "on" or "off" in response to nutrition, stress, sleep patterns, emotions, toxins, physical activity, and lifestyle choices. In simple language, genes are like switches, and daily life determines which switches are flipped.

A familiar example makes this clear: consider a smartphone that comes with many features—camera, navigation, internet, power-saving mode, and security systems. All these features exist in the phone from the beginning, but only certain functions are active at a given time depending on how the phone is used. If the phone is constantly overheated, poorly charged, and overloaded with unnecessary apps, its performance declines despite having a perfect original design. Similarly, the human body may have an excellent genetic blueprint, but poor lifestyle "usage" can suppress beneficial genes and activate harmful pathways. Thus, health or disease reflects not just what genes one has, but how those genes are used.

Ayurveda described this hereditary intelligence long before the discovery of DNA through the concepts of **Beeja**, **Beejabhaga**, and **Beejabhagavayava**. Beeja represents the fundamental reproductive seed inherited from parents, comparable to the genetic material. Beejabhaga refers to specific parts of that seed responsible for forming organs and systems, while Beejabhagavayava represents even finer subdivisions governing subtle traits and functions. Classical Ayurvedic texts clearly recognized that while structural potential is determined at conception, the final outcome depends on multiple factors, including parental health, maternal nutrition, mental state, age, and environment during pregnancy. This understanding is remarkably aligned with modern concepts of prenatal epigenetics and developmental programming.

"Beejabhāga doṣāt garbhavikṛtiḥ"

Defects in hereditary components cause congenital disorders

— *Charaka Samhita*

In simple terms, Ayurveda acknowledged that defects or disturbances at the level of the blueprint can produce congenital abnormalities, but it also emphasized that many disorders arise not from defective seeds, but from improper nourishment and care of the developing system. Modern research now confirms that maternal stress, poor nutrition, toxin exposure, and metabolic imbalance during pregnancy can alter gene expression in the fetus, increasing the risk of diabetes, obesity, cardiovascular disease, and mental health disorders later in life—even when DNA itself is normal.

The most important implication of this understanding is that genes are not destiny. While certain genetic predispositions exist, they do not guarantee disease. A person may carry genes associated with diabetes or heart disease, yet never develop these conditions if lifestyle supports healthy gene expression. Conversely, someone with no strong genetic risk may still develop chronic disease due to persistent stress, poor diet, sleep deprivation, and toxic exposures. Disease, therefore, often reflects mismanagement of genetic potential rather than genetic deficiency itself.

From an engineering perspective, this is a powerful and hopeful insight. It means the blueprint is robust, adaptable, and forgiving—but not invincible. When the operating conditions respect design limits, the system performs optimally. When they do not, even the best design suffers. Ayurveda recognized this long ago and emphasized right conduct, right diet, and right living as essential tools for protecting hereditary intelligence. Modern epigenetics now validates this ancient wisdom, confirming that while we cannot change the blueprint we inherit, we can profoundly influence how it is expressed.

1.4 Energy Engineering: Agni and Metabolic Intelligence

No engine—no matter how perfectly designed—can function without a reliable and well-regulated energy system. The human body possesses the most efficient and adaptable energy-production system known to science. At the cellular level, energy is generated in the form of ATP within mitochondria, tiny structures often described as cellular power plants. These mitochondria convert nutrients derived from food and oxygen from breathing into usable energy that powers every biological activity, from heartbeat and muscle movement to thinking, immunity, and tissue repair. What makes this system remarkable is not only its efficiency, but its ability to operate continuously, adjusting output minute by minute according to the body's needs.

A key feature that distinguishes human bio-energy from mechanical engines is **metabolic flexibility**. Machines usually operate on a single fuel type and fail or lose efficiency when that fuel changes. The human body, in contrast, can shift smoothly between multiple fuel sources—glucose after meals, fatty acids during fasting, and ketone bodies during prolonged energy demand or scarcity. This flexibility allows survival during feast and famine, rest and exertion, illness and recovery. Modern medical science now recognizes that loss of this flexibility is a central defect in many chronic diseases. When the body becomes locked into inefficient energy use—such as constant dependence on glucose with impaired fat utilization—conditions like obesity, type 2 diabetes, fatty liver disease, cardiovascular disorders, cancer, and neurodegeneration begin to develop. In simple terms, the engine still has fuel, but it can no longer use it properly.

Ayurveda described this entire energy economy through the concept of **Agni**, a term often translated as "digestive fire," but whose meaning is far broader. Agni represents the intelligence that governs all transformation in the body—digestion of food, metabolism of nutrients, cellular energy production, tissue nourishment, and even mental processing. Charaka Samhita states clearly:

"Agniḥ sarva śarīrāṇāṃ mūlaṃ"
Agni is the root of all bodily functions

This statement reflects an engineering truth: energy transformation is the foundation of all performance. When Agni functions optimally, food is digested efficiently, nutrients are converted into usable energy, tissues are nourished properly, immunity remains strong, and the mind stays clear and alert. When Agni is weak, irregular, or overloaded, the same food fails to nourish. Instead, it produces **Ama**, a toxic metabolic residue that clogs pathways, interferes with cellular communication, and triggers inflammation. Modern science describes similar processes as incomplete metabolism, oxidative stress, mitochondrial dysfunction, and chronic low-grade inflammation.

A simple example helps clarify this concept. Two people eat the same meal. One feels light, energized, and satisfied; the other feels heavy, sleepy, bloated, or irritable. The food is identical, yet the outcome is different. The difference lies not in calories or nutrients alone, but in how effectively each person's metabolic engine processes that food. Ayurveda would say one person has balanced Agni, while the other has impaired Agni. Modern medicine would describe this as differences in insulin sensitivity, mitochondrial efficiency, gut health, and inflammatory state. Both explanations point to the same underlying reality: energy management determines health.

Another analogy is that of fire used for cooking. A well-controlled flame cooks food evenly and efficiently. A weak flame leaves food undercooked, while an excessively strong flame burns it. Similarly, balanced Agni transforms food into nourishment. Weak Agni leaves digestion incomplete, producing Ama. Excessive or unstable Agni leads to burning, inflammation, acidity, and tissue damage. Thus, health depends not on how much food is eaten, but on how intelligently it is transformed.

Understanding Agni as metabolic intelligence also explains why simply increasing food intake or taking supplements does not automatically improve energy. Many people with fatigue eat more or consume stimulants, yet remain tired. From an engineering perspective, this is like pouring more fuel into an engine with a faulty combustion system. Without correcting the transformation process, additional input only increases waste and stress. Ayurveda, therefore, emphasized correcting Agni before focusing on nourishment—a principle now echoed in modern approaches that prioritize metabolic health, gut function, and mitochondrial support.

In essence, energy engineering in the human body is not about fuel quantity but about fuel intelligence. The body is rarely energy-deficient; it is often energy-mismanaged. Agni represents the wisdom that decides how energy is extracted, distributed, and used. Preserving this metabolic intelligence is central to preventing disease, maintaining vitality, and sustaining long-term health.

1.5 Control Systems: Regulation Before Structure

Energy alone does not guarantee efficient performance; without regulation, even the most powerful engine becomes unstable and destructive. In all advanced engineering systems, control mechanisms and feedback loops are essential to maintain balance, precision, and safety. The human body represents the most sophisticated regulatory architecture ever observed, integrating neural signals, hormonal communication, immune responses, and autonomic control into a single, intelligent system that operates continuously without conscious supervision. This regulatory intelligence allows the body to maintain internal stability despite constant changes in environment, activity, emotional state, and energy availability.

At the center of this control network lies the brain, functioning as a highly efficient central processor. Unlike artificial processors that require massive energy input and external programming, the brain consumes minimal energy while performing complex tasks such as prediction, emotional regulation, learning, creativity, decision-making, and self-awareness. It constantly receives information from internal organs and the external environment, compares current conditions with stored experience, predicts outcomes, and sends corrective commands through nerves and hormones. Alongside the brain, the autonomic nervous system quietly manages essential life processes—heart rate, blood pressure, breathing, digestion, body temperature, and glandular secretion—without conscious effort. Hormones act as long-range messengers, coordinating growth, metabolism, stress response, reproduction, and repair over longer time scales. Immune signaling adds another layer of regulation, continuously surveying the body, removing damaged cells, and coordinating healing responses.

Modern medicine now increasingly recognizes that many chronic diseases arise not from sudden injury or irreversible damage, but from long-standing failure of regulatory control. Conditions such as hypertension, type 2 diabetes, irritable bowel syndrome, anxiety disorders, autoimmune diseases, and neurodegenerative disorders often develop silently over the years. During this long period, organs may appear structurally normal on scans and tests, yet regulatory balance is already compromised. Blood pressure fluctuates abnormally, glucose regulation becomes inefficient, gut-brain communication is disturbed, immune responses become misdirected, and stress responses remain persistently activated. Structural damage appears only later, when the capacity for regulation and repair has been exhausted. This explains why treating only organs without addressing regulation often leads to incomplete or temporary relief.

Ayurveda recognized this principle long before the discovery of nerves, hormones, and immune pathways. It identified **Vata Dosha** as the master regulator of the body's internal control systems.

> **"Vātādṛte nāsti kriyā"**
> *No bodily function occurs without Vata*
>
> — *Charaka Samhita*

Vata governs all movement and communication within the body—nerve impulses, circulation of blood, respiration, initiation of digestion, elimination of waste, muscle activity, and mental processes such as alertness and adaptability. In simple terms, Vata is like the wiring, software, and signal transmission system of a complex machine. Even if all components are structurally intact, faulty wiring leads to malfunction. When Vata is balanced, regulation is smooth and adaptive. When Vata is disturbed—by chronic stress, irregular daily routines, insufficient sleep, excessive sensory stimulation, or erratic eating patterns—control begins to fail.

A layman's example illustrates this clearly. Imagine a house with excellent construction but unstable electrical wiring. Lights flicker, appliances malfunction, and power surges damage equipment over time. The structure of the house may remain intact initially, but repeated electrical instability eventually causes fires or breakdown. Similarly, in the human body, Vata disturbance first causes functional symptoms such as anxiety, insomnia, palpitations, bloating, constipation, variable appetite, and fatigue. If ignored, these functional disturbances progress to metabolic disorders, inflammation, and eventually structural disease such as hypertension, arthritis, neurodegeneration, or organ failure.

This understanding highlights a crucial engineering truth: regulation must be restored before structure can be preserved. Treating high blood pressure without addressing stress and autonomic imbalance, or managing blood sugar without correcting nervous system overload, is like reinforcing walls while ignoring unstable control systems. Ayurveda therefore emphasized regular routines, adequate rest, rhythmic eating, mental calmness, and grounding practices to stabilize Vata and protect the body's regulatory intelligence. Modern science now confirms that restoring nervous system balance, circadian rhythm, and stress regulation is foundational for preventing and reversing chronic disease.

1.6 Waste Management: Internal Sanitation Determines Longevity

Every functioning system, no matter how advanced, inevitably produces waste. In engineering, efficient waste disposal is considered just as important as energy supply or control mechanisms. If waste is not removed regularly, it accumulates, interferes with function, increases wear, and ultimately leads to system failure. The human body follows this same fundamental principle. It is equipped with a highly sophisticated, multi-organ waste-management network that operates continuously to maintain internal cleanliness and protect long-term function. This network includes the lungs, kidneys, liver, gastrointestinal tract, and skin, each performing specialized elimination roles that together preserve internal balance.

The lungs remove carbon dioxide, a waste product of cellular respiration. Even small increases in carbon dioxide disturb blood chemistry and brain function, showing how sensitive the system is to waste retention. The kidneys filter blood continuously, removing nitrogenous waste, excess salts, acids, and toxins while maintaining fluid and electrolyte balance. The liver acts as the central detoxification and recycling unit, transforming harmful substances into forms that can be safely eliminated through bile or urine. The gut removes undigested food, microbial waste, and bile pigments, while the skin eliminates water, salts, and minor toxins through sweat. When these systems function efficiently, waste is cleared before it can harm tissues. When they are overloaded or impaired, waste accumulates silently and gradually disrupts multiple systems.

Ayurveda recognized the central importance of elimination and expressed it clearly:

> **"Mala dhāraṇāt rogāḥ jāyante"**
> *Retention of waste causes disease*
>
> — *Ashtanga Hridaya*

This statement reflects a simple but powerful truth: health depends not only on what the body takes in, but equally on what it can eliminate. Ayurveda described three primary wastes—**Purisha** (feces), **Mutra** (urine), and **Sweda** (sweat)—and emphasized that improper formation or elimination of any of these initiates disease. Beyond normal waste, Ayurveda identified **Ama**, a toxic, sticky residue formed when digestion and metabolism are incomplete. Unlike ordinary waste, Ama circulates within the body, obstructing channels (**Srotorodha**) and interfering with cellular communication. Modern science now recognizes similar processes in the form of oxidative stress, inflammatory mediators, metabolic endotoxins, endothelial dysfunction, and gut dysbiosis.

A simple analogy makes this concept easy to understand. Consider a city with an excellent water supply and power grid, but a failing garbage collection system. Even with abundant resources, the city becomes unhealthy as waste piles up, attracts pests, spreads infection, and blocks normal activity. Similarly, a person may eat nutritious food and take appropriate medicines, yet still feel unwell if waste is not eliminated properly. Constipation, poor sweating, shallow breathing, or impaired liver detoxification allow toxins to accumulate, leading to fatigue, headaches, skin problems, joint pain, hormonal imbalance, and chronic inflammation. In such cases, adding more supplements or medications is like delivering more goods to a city whose garbage system is already blocked.

From an engineering perspective, waste accumulation increases internal resistance and reduces efficiency. In the body, this manifests as sluggish metabolism, reduced energy, immune dysfunction, and accelerated aging. Modern medicine now acknowledges that impaired detoxification and elimination contribute to diseases such as gout (uric acid retention), atherosclerosis (lipid and inflammatory waste deposition), fatty liver disease, autoimmune disorders, and neurodegeneration. Ayurveda recognized these outcomes long ago and emphasized therapies that restore elimination—such as proper hydration, dietary regulation, sweating therapies, bowel regulation, and cleansing procedures—to clear Ama and reopen channels.

The engine analogy captures this principle perfectly. Even the most advanced engine will fail if its exhaust system is blocked. Back pressure builds, combustion becomes inefficient, parts overheat, and breakdown follows. In the human body, blocked elimination pathways create a similar internal back pressure, disrupting circulation, metabolism, and communication. Longevity, therefore, is not determined solely by nutrition or genetics, but by the efficiency of internal sanitation. A clean system runs smoothly, ages slowly, and resists disease.

1.7 Self-Repair and Regeneration: Rasayana and Repair Intelligence

One of the most remarkable features of the human body, and the clearest evidence of its superior engineering, is its built-in capacity for self-repair. Unlike machines that require external technicians and replacement parts, the human body carries its own repair intelligence within every tissue. Stem cells continuously regenerate skin, blood, and gut lining. Immune cells identify and remove damaged or abnormal cells. DNA repair enzymes correct errors that occur during cell division or due to environmental stress. Structural proteins such as collagen are constantly broken down and rebuilt to maintain strength and flexibility. Modern science now understands aging not as a sudden breakdown, but as a gradual decline in the efficiency and coordination of these repair mechanisms. When repair keeps pace with damage, health is maintained; when repair falls behind, degeneration and disease begin.

Ayurveda recognized this principle thousands of years ago and organized it into a complete medical discipline known as **Rasayana**.

> **"Rasāyanaṃ vayasthāpanam"**
> *Rasayana preserves youth and delays aging*
>
> — *Charaka Samhita*

Rasayana does not promise immortality; instead, it aims to preserve the body's natural capacity to repair, regenerate, and adapt. In simple terms, Rasayana therapies strengthen the body's "maintenance department." They nourish tissues at a deep level, enhance immunity (Ojas), improve metabolic efficiency, and protect against premature degeneration. From an engineering viewpoint, Rasayana is preventive maintenance that sustains the efficiency of repair systems rather than emergency repair after failure.

A simple example helps illustrate this concept. Imagine two identical houses exposed to the same weather conditions. In one house, small cracks are repaired early, paint is refreshed, leaks are fixed, and wiring is maintained. In the other, minor damage is ignored. Over time, the first house remains strong and functional, while the second deteriorates rapidly. The difference lies not in exposure to damage, but in timely repair. Similarly, all human bodies experience daily wear from metabolism, stress, and environmental exposure. Longevity depends on how efficiently this wear is repaired.

Modern research increasingly validates the Ayurvedic concept of Rasayana. Studies show that many Rasayana herbs and practices have antioxidant properties that reduce oxidative damage, immunomodulatory effects that improve immune balance, and neuroprotective actions that preserve brain function. Some enhance mitochondrial function, supporting cellular energy and repair, while others influence stem cell activity and tissue regeneration. These effects align closely with modern understanding of aging as a failure of repair and regeneration rather than simple passage of time.

Another everyday example clarifies this idea further. Consider muscle growth after exercise. Exercise causes microscopic damage to muscle fibers. If the body repairs this damage efficiently through rest, nutrition, and hormonal balance, muscles become stronger. If repair is inadequate due to poor sleep, stress, or malnutrition, weakness and injury develop. Damage itself is not harmful; failure to repair is. Rasayana works on the same principle at the whole-body level, ensuring that repair keeps pace with daily damage.

In practical terms, this understanding shifts the focus of healthcare. Instead of obsessing over avoiding all stress or damage—an impossible task—true longevity medicine aims to preserve repair intelligence. Adequate sleep, proper digestion, balanced metabolism, emotional stability, and Rasayana support all contribute to maintaining this internal repair capacity. When repair systems remain strong, the body can tolerate stress, heal injuries, resist disease, and age gracefully. Thus, longevity is not achieved by eliminating damage, but by sustaining the body's extraordinary ability to repair itself.

1.8 Early Warning Systems: Disease Is Never Sudden

All advanced engineering systems are designed with early warning and predictive maintenance mechanisms. Sensors detect small deviations in temperature, pressure, vibration, or efficiency long before a breakdown occurs. These warnings allow engineers to intervene early, preventing costly and irreversible damage. The human body follows the same intelligent principle. It continuously monitors its own internal state and sends warning signals whenever the balance is disturbed. Fatigue, unexplained pain, disturbed sleep, digestive discomfort, mood changes, reduced stamina, and declining motivation are not random complaints or minor inconveniences; they are the body's built-in alert system indicating that something is going wrong at the functional level.

Ayurveda described this predictive intelligence with remarkable precision through the concepts of **Purvarupa** (early warning signs) and **Shatkriyakala** (six stages of disease development). According to this model, disease does not appear suddenly or without warning. It progresses through predictable stages, beginning with subtle imbalance and ending in full structural pathology if corrective action is not taken. In the early stages, the process is completely reversible through simple measures such as dietary correction, lifestyle regulation, and restoration of digestion and sleep. However, when early warnings are ignored, the imbalance deepens, spreads to tissues, and eventually manifests as an established disease that requires intensive treatment.

A simple example makes this clear. Before a wall develops deep cracks, there are small signs—hairline fractures, damp patches, or peeling paint. If these early signs are addressed, major damage is prevented. If they are ignored, the structure weakens, and repair becomes expensive and difficult. Similarly, before diabetes develops, the body signals rising fatigue, increased thirst, weight changes, and sugar cravings. Before heart disease, there may be poor sleep, stress intolerance, indigestion, and reduced exercise capacity. Before arthritis, there is stiffness, mild pain, and reduced flexibility. These early signals are opportunities for correction, not problems to be suppressed.

Modern medical science now strongly supports this ancient understanding. Biomarkers reveal that a disease begins long before diagnosis. Prediabetes precedes diabetes by many years, during which blood sugar regulation is impaired but still reversible. Chronic low-grade inflammation, detectable through markers such as CRP, exists years before heart attacks or strokes occur. Neurodegenerative diseases like Alzheimer's begin with subtle cognitive changes and metabolic alterations decades before memory loss becomes obvious. These findings confirm a crucial truth: by the time a disease is named, it has already been present for a long time at a functional level.

From an engineering perspective, ignoring early warnings is the fastest way to guarantee failure. Yet modern culture often does exactly this with the human body. Fatigue is masked with stimulants, pain with analgesics, sleep problems with sedatives, and digestive issues with temporary relief measures. While symptoms may temporarily disappear, the underlying imbalance continues to progress. Ayurveda cautioned against this approach, emphasizing that suppressing warning signals without correcting their cause accelerates disease rather than preventing it.

Understanding disease as ignored feedback changes the entire approach to health. Instead of asking, "What medicine will remove this symptom?" the more intelligent question becomes, "What is the body trying to tell me?" When early warning signs are respected and addressed, the body's natural self-correcting mechanisms restore balance. When they are ignored, the system is forced to escalate the signal in the form of more severe symptoms and structural damage. Disease, therefore, is never sudden. It is the final stage of a long conversation between the body and the individual—one that was repeatedly ignored.

1.9 Disease as Engineering Failure, Not Enemy

One of the most persistent misunderstandings in modern healthcare is the tendency to view disease as an enemy that must be fought and eliminated. From an engineering perspective, this mindset is fundamentally flawed. In complex systems, failure is rarely caused by an external enemy; it results from internal imbalance, overload, misuse, or breakdown of regulation. The human body follows the same logic. Fever, inflammation, pain, altered metabolism, and fatigue are not acts of betrayal by the body. They are adaptive responses—protective signals generated by an intelligent system attempting to restore balance. Treating these responses as enemies and suppressing them without understanding their cause is equivalent to disabling warning systems in a machine while allowing internal damage to continue.

A simple example helps clarify this idea. Imagine a factory where an alarm sounds because a machine is overheating. The alarm is not the problem; it is a signal that cooling is inadequate or load is excessive. If the alarm is silenced without reducing the load or improving cooling, the machine will eventually fail catastrophically. Similarly, fever raises body temperature to slow down pathogens and enhance immune activity, inflammation increases blood flow and repair processes, and pain restricts movement to prevent further injury. When these responses are suppressed without addressing the underlying imbalance—such as infection, stress, poor digestion, or overload—the body loses its ability to signal danger, and disease progresses silently.

Ayurveda understood disease as a disturbance of balance rather than an invasion by an enemy. Its primary therapeutic goal was not to attack symptoms but to restore harmony among regulatory forces, metabolism, tissues, elimination, and mind. This approach recognizes that the body is fundamentally intelligent and self-healing when supported correctly. For example, inflammation in a joint is not merely a nuisance to be suppressed; it reflects overuse, improper mechanics, poor circulation, or metabolic waste accumulation. Addressing these causes allows inflammation to resolve naturally, whereas repeated suppression may provide temporary relief but accelerates degeneration.

Modern systems medicine is now rediscovering this perspective. Research shows that chronic suppression of adaptive responses can worsen long-term outcomes. Overuse of anti-inflammatory drugs can impair tissue repair and damage organs. Excessive suppression of fever may prolong infections. Aggressive glucose-lowering without addressing insulin resistance can increase complications. These findings reinforce the idea that symptoms are not the disease itself, but expressions of deeper system failure. Treating only the symptom is like fixing the paint on a cracked wall without reinforcing the foundation.

Understanding disease as an engineering failure shifts responsibility and empowerment back to the individual and clinician. Instead of asking, "How do we destroy this disease?" the question becomes, "What system has failed, and why?" This approach encourages early correction, lifestyle adjustment, metabolic repair, and stress regulation—interventions that restore system integrity rather than fight the body. Ayurveda emphasized this balance-restoration model centuries ago, and modern systems biology is now moving in the same direction. When disease is understood as feedback rather than an enemy, medicine becomes preventive, rational, and truly healing.

1.10 Health Redefined: Efficiency, Not Absence of Disease

Health is often misunderstood as simply the absence of a diagnosed disease. If medical reports appear normal and no major illness has been identified, a person is commonly labeled as "healthy." From an engineering perspective, however, this definition is incomplete and misleading. In complex systems, the absence of visible failure does not guarantee optimal performance. A machine may still be running, yet operating inefficiently, consuming excess fuel, overheating, or wearing out prematurely. Similarly, a human body may have normal laboratory values and imaging studies, yet function far below its true potential. True health is better defined as **system efficiency**—the ability of the body to perform its functions smoothly, economically, and adaptively over time.

From this viewpoint, health includes stable energy throughout the day without dependence on stimulants, metabolic flexibility that allows the body to handle different foods and fasting without distress, clear and focused cognition, emotional stability, strong immunity, efficient digestion and elimination, and structural integrity of muscles, joints, and organs. It also includes adaptive resilience—the capacity to recover quickly from stress, illness, injury, or exertion. A healthy system absorbs shocks and returns to balance, just as a well-designed engine tolerates load variations without damage. When these qualities are present, disease struggles to establish itself, even in the presence of environmental challenges.

Ayurveda defined health with remarkable precision in a way that closely mirrors this engineering concept:

> **"Sama doṣaḥ samāgniś ca sama dhātu mala kriyāḥ**
> **Prasanna ātmendriya manaḥ svastha ity abhidhīyate."**
>
> — *Sushruta Samhita*

This definition states that health exists when regulatory forces (Dosha) are balanced, metabolism (Agni) functions properly, tissues (Dhatu) are well maintained, waste elimination (Mala) is efficient, and the mind and senses are calm and clear. In simple language, this means that all systems are working in coordination, without excessive strain or deficiency. Health is not just physical strength or absence of pain; it includes mental clarity, emotional stability, and efficient internal functioning.

A Simple example illustrates this difference clearly. Two people may both be free from diagnosed disease. One wakes up refreshed, digests food comfortably, maintains steady energy, handles stress calmly, and recovers quickly from illness or exertion. The other feels tired despite rest, experiences frequent indigestion, mood swings, and recurrent minor infections, yet has "normal" reports. By conventional definitions, both are healthy. From an engineering perspective, however, the first person's system is efficient, while the second is operating with hidden inefficiencies that, if uncorrected, will eventually lead to disease.

Modern systems biology increasingly supports this expanded definition of health. It emphasizes resilience, adaptability, and network efficiency rather than isolated organ function. Researchers now study heart rate variability as a marker of autonomic flexibility, metabolic markers of fuel adaptability, inflammatory markers as indicators of system stress, and cognitive measures of mental efficiency. These parameters often change long before disease is diagnosed, reinforcing the idea that health and disease exist on a continuum rather than as opposites.

Redefining health in this way transforms medical practice and personal responsibility. Instead of waiting for disease to appear, the focus shifts toward optimizing daily function, restoring balance, and maintaining efficiency. Ayurveda adopted this approach thousands of years ago by prioritizing the protection of the healthy individual as the first duty of medicine. When health is understood as efficiency rather than mere survival, prevention becomes practical, measurable, and meaningful.

Chapter 2

Blueprint of the Human Machine: Understanding the Design Before Repair

2.1 Introduction: Why Every Repair Begins With a Blueprint

In every field of engineering, a blueprint is the foundation of all repair and maintenance work. Whether an engineer is fixing a car engine, repairing an electrical circuit, strengthening a bridge, or correcting a software error, the first step is always to understand the original design of the system. The blueprint explains not only where each part is located, but also why that part exists, how it communicates with other parts, how energy or information flows through the system, and what limits the system is designed to tolerate. When this understanding is missing, repairs become guesswork. The system may seem to work temporarily, but hidden damage continues beneath the surface, leading to repeated failures and eventually complete breakdown.

A simple example can be seen in everyday vehicle repair. If a car repeatedly overheats, simply adding water to the radiator may cool the engine for a short time. However, without understanding the blueprint of the cooling system—such as a faulty thermostat, blocked radiator, or damaged water pump—the overheating will return and may ultimately damage the engine beyond repair. True repair requires knowledge of how the entire system is designed to manage heat, not just temporary symptom control. This same engineering principle applies to all complex systems.

The human body follows this law even more strictly than machines. Unlike a car or a computer, the human body cannot be turned off, opened fully, or replaced part by part without consequences. It is a living, self-operating system that works continuously from the moment of conception until death. Every second, millions of processes—breathing, circulation, digestion, nerve signaling, hormone release, and immune defense—occur simultaneously without conscious effort. Treating disease without understanding this design is like trying to fix a flying airplane without knowing its internal structure or control systems. The risk of repeated failure is extremely high.

For example, consider a person who frequently experiences acidity or indigestion. Taking an antacid may give immediate relief, just as silencing a warning alarm reduces noise. However, without understanding the blueprint of digestion—how food is processed, how acid is regulated, how nerves control stomach movement, and how lifestyle affects digestion—the problem keeps returning. Over time, this repeated neglect may lead to ulcers, nutrient deficiency, or metabolic disease. The symptom was treated, but the design principle was ignored.

Another clear example is high blood pressure. Many people believe that blood pressure itself is the disease. Medicines may lower the numbers temporarily, but if the blueprint is not understood—such as how stress, sleep, salt intake, emotional strain, and nervous system balance regulate blood pressure—the condition often worsens over time. This is similar to tightening bolts on a machine that is under excessive load without reducing the load itself. Eventually, parts begin to fail despite repeated adjustments.

Modern lifestyle diseases provide strong evidence that ignoring the blueprint leads to chronic problems. Conditions such as diabetes, obesity, joint pain, anxiety, and heart disease do not appear suddenly. They develop slowly as the body is repeatedly pushed beyond its design limits—wrong food, irregular sleep, constant stress, lack of movement, and emotional overload. When treatment begins only after the disease is diagnosed, the system is already damaged. The body's early warning signals were present for years but were ignored or suppressed.

The human body also differs from machines in one crucial way: it has built-in intelligence and self-repair ability. A machine does not heal itself; it waits for an external technician. The body continuously repairs damaged cells, adjusts hormone levels, strengthens immunity, and adapts to stress. However, this intelligence functions properly only when the system operates according to its blueprint. When design rules are repeatedly violated, self-repair becomes inefficient, and disease gradually replaces health.

Therefore, understanding the blueprint of the human body is not optional—it is essential. Without this understanding, medical treatment becomes reactive rather than preventive, temporary rather than lasting. Just as no engineer would repair a complex machine without studying its design, no healthcare approach can truly succeed without respecting the original design logic of the human body. Health is not achieved by fighting disease alone, but by maintaining harmony with the blueprint that governs how the human machine is built to function.

2.2 The Human Body as a Designed Biological System

Modern biology no longer views the human body as a random collection of chemicals reacting by chance. Scientific research in genetics, systems biology, neuroscience, and physiology has clearly shown that the body is an **intelligently organized system with a clear design logic**. Every organ is built with a specific structure suited to its function, just as different parts of a machine are shaped according to their role. For example, the lungs have millions of tiny air sacs to maximize oxygen exchange, the heart has strong muscular walls to pump blood continuously, and the kidneys are designed with fine filters to clean the blood without losing essential substances. These structures are not accidental; they reflect purposeful engineering.

At a deeper level, the body works in a **hierarchical and step-by-step manner**. Simple molecules form cells, cells form tissues, tissues form organs, and organs work together as systems. Biochemical pathways follow strict sequences, much like steps in a factory assembly line. If one step is skipped or rushed, the final product becomes faulty. For instance, digestion occurs in a specific order—from the mouth to the stomach to the intestines. When this sequence is disturbed by overeating, eating at odd hours, or eating incompatible foods, the entire system suffers. This explains why irregular habits cause problems such as acidity, bloating, or fatigue long before serious disease develops.

The human body is also **modular**, meaning it is organized into systems such as the digestive system, respiratory system, nervous system, endocrine system, and immune system. Each system has its own role, yet none works in isolation. Just as in a large building where electrical, plumbing, and ventilation systems must work together, the body's systems constantly communicate. For example, chronic stress affects the nervous system, which then alters hormones, digestion, immunity, and even blood pressure. Treating only one system without understanding its interaction with others often leads to incomplete or temporary relief.

Another remarkable design feature of the human body is **redundancy**, or built-in backup systems. In engineering, critical systems always have backups to prevent total failure. Similarly, humans have two kidneys, two lungs, paired arteries, and overlapping hormone systems. Even at the cellular level, multiple pathways exist to produce energy. This is why a person can live a normal life with one kidney or one lung. Disease becomes visible only when damage exceeds this reserve capacity. This explains why people often feel "fine" for years before suddenly being diagnosed with a serious illness—the backups were quietly compensating until they were exhausted.

The body also relies heavily on **feedback loops**, which allow constant self-correction. Blood sugar, body temperature, blood pressure, and oxygen levels are continuously monitored and adjusted automatically. If blood sugar rises, insulin is released; if body temperature increases, sweating begins. These processes happen without conscious effort. When feedback loops fail or are repeatedly overloaded, disease develops. For example, in diabetes, the blood sugar regulation loop becomes inefficient due to long-term overload. Treating sugar levels alone without restoring the feedback system results in lifelong dependence on medication.

Equally important are the body's **predictive warning signals**, which act like dashboard indicators in a vehicle. Pain, fatigue, hunger, thirst, sleepiness, anxiety, and low mood are not diseases by themselves—they are early messages that something is out of balance. Ignoring these signals is like covering the warning lights on a car dashboard. For instance, chronic fatigue is often an early sign of poor sleep, nutritional deficiency, stress overload, or hormonal imbalance. Suppressing fatigue with stimulants may allow temporary functioning, but worsens long-term damage.

From an engineering standpoint, the human body is far superior to any machine because it does not merely operate—it **adapts, learns, repairs, and anticipates future needs**. Muscles grow stronger with use, immunity improves after exposure, and the brain rewires itself through learning. No machine can improve its own design through experience the way the human body does. However, this intelligence works best only when the system is respected and supported, not forced beyond its limits.

Despite this, modern healthcare often intervenes only after visible failure occurs. Medical attention usually begins when blood reports are abnormal, scans show damage, or symptoms become severe. At this stage, the system has already crossed safe design limits. Treatment then focuses on suppressing symptoms, correcting numbers, or replacing damaged parts. While this approach is essential in emergencies—such as trauma, infections, or organ failure—it often overlooks the deeper question of why the body's intelligent design failed to protect itself earlier.

For example, joint replacement surgery can restore mobility, but it does not explain why cartilage wore out prematurely. Heart bypass surgery can save life, but it does not correct years of metabolic stress, poor sleep, emotional strain, and lifestyle overload that led to vessel damage. Similarly, long-term medication may control symptoms but may not restore the body's lost self-regulation. Without understanding the body as a designed biological system, treatment remains reactive rather than preventive.

Therefore, true healthcare must begin with respect for the body's design. When treatment aligns with the body's natural architecture, feedback systems, and adaptive intelligence, healing becomes deeper and more sustainable. Understanding *why* the system failed is far more powerful than merely fixing *what* has broken. This shift—from crisis repair to design-based care—is essential for preventing chronic disease and preserving long-term health.

2.3 Modern Medicine and Late-Stage Repairs

Most chronic diseases do not appear suddenly or without warning. They develop slowly over many years as the body is repeatedly pushed away from its original design principles. The human body is built to adapt and compensate, so early damage is often hidden. During this long, silent phase, the body uses its reserve capacity and backup systems to maintain outward normality. By the time a disease is diagnosed, the system has usually been under strain for a very long time. In simple terms, modern medicine often meets the disease at the end of the story, not at the beginning.

Type 2 diabetes is a clear example of late-stage repair. Long before blood sugar rises, the body struggles with excess calorie intake, irregular meals, lack of physical activity, poor sleep, and chronic stress. To cope, the pancreas releases more insulin, and the cells gradually become less responsive to it. This phase may last for years without obvious symptoms. When diabetes is finally diagnosed, treatment focuses mainly on lowering blood sugar numbers. While this is important for immediate safety, it does not correct the deeper problem—the body's reduced ability to process and use energy efficiently. It is similar to reducing smoke from a factory chimney without fixing the faulty machinery producing the smoke.

High blood pressure offers another simple illustration. Blood pressure often rises as a protective response to long-term stress, stiff blood vessels, poor sleep, emotional strain, excess salt, and lack of physical activity. The body increases pressure to maintain blood flow to vital organs. When treatment targets only the pressure reading, the underlying causes—such as nervous system overactivity and vessel damage—remain unchanged. This is like increasing the strength of a water pump without repairing the narrowed pipes. Over time, the strain damages the heart, kidneys, eyes, and brain, even though the numbers may look controlled.

Osteoarthritis clearly demonstrates how late-stage repairs ignore early warning signals. Joint pain and stiffness often begin years before X-rays show damage. Poor posture, improper walking patterns, obesity, nutritional deficiencies, and low muscle strength slowly overload the joint. The cartilage, which has very limited healing capacity, gradually thins. When pain becomes severe and movement is restricted, joint replacement is performed. While surgery can restore mobility, it does not correct faulty movement patterns or metabolic inflammation. As a result, other joints often begin to fail later. This is comparable to replacing worn-out tires without correcting wheel alignment—the problem simply shifts elsewhere.

Neurodegenerative diseases such as Alzheimer's and Parkinson's represent some of the most extreme examples of late-stage intervention. Memory loss, tremors, or movement difficulties appear only after a large number of nerve cells have already died. Years earlier, subtle problems may have been present—poor sleep, chronic stress, digestive disturbances, mood changes, or long-standing inflammation. These early signals are often dismissed as normal aging or lifestyle issues. By the time the disease is diagnosed, treatment can only slow progression, not restore lost brain tissue. This is like repairing a building after a major structural collapse rather than strengthening it when small cracks first appeared.

Heart disease follows a similar pattern. Cholesterol buildup and vessel damage develop silently over decades due to poor diet, stress, smoking, lack of exercise, and disturbed sleep. Chest pain or a heart attack occurs only when the blockage becomes critical. Emergency treatments such as stents or bypass surgery save lives, but they address the blocked vessel, not the long-term lifestyle and metabolic causes that created the blockage. Without correcting these deeper issues, new blockages often develop elsewhere.

In engineering terms, these medical interventions are **late-stage repairs**. They are performed after repeated violations of the body's blueprint—wrong fuel, excessive load, ignored warning signals, and delayed maintenance. Such repairs are necessary and often lifesaving, but they are not true solutions. They do not restore the original design intelligence of the system; they merely prevent immediate failure.

A truly effective healthcare approach must therefore shift its focus earlier. Instead of waiting for breakdown, it must recognize early signals, reduce overload, restore balance, and support the body's natural self-repair mechanisms. Just as a well-maintained machine lasts longer and performs better, a body that is cared for according to its design principles can avoid many chronic diseases. Understanding disease as a late-stage outcome rather than a sudden event is the first step toward preventive, intelligent, and sustainable health care.

2.4 Ayurveda: Medicine Built on Blueprint Knowledge

Ayurveda was founded on the principle that effective treatment is impossible without understanding the body's original design. Classical Ayurvedic texts repeatedly emphasize that a physician must first understand how the body is built and how it functions before attempting to correct disease. For this reason, a detailed study of **Sharira Rachana** (body structure) and **Sharira Kriya** (body function) was considered essential training for every practitioner. Disease was never viewed as an isolated problem of one organ, but as a disturbance in the coordinated working of the whole system. This approach is similar to systems engineering, where failure in one component is always traced back to the interaction between multiple subsystems.

Unlike modern medicine, which often focuses on individual organs, Ayurveda viewed the body as a **single integrated network** governed by regulatory principles. The concept of **Dosha** explains how movement, transformation, and stability are controlled throughout the body. Vata governs movement and communication, Pitta governs transformation and metabolism, and Kapha governs structure and lubrication. These are not substances but functional principles, much like control algorithms in engineering. For example, joint stiffness, dry skin, constipation, and anxiety often occur together because they share the same disturbed regulatory principle, not because each problem is separate. Treating the regulation restores multiple symptoms at once.

The concept of **Agni**, or metabolic intelligence, lies at the heart of the Ayurvedic blueprint. Agni does not refer only to stomach digestion;

it represents the body's ability to transform food into energy, tissues, and vitality at every level. When Agni is strong, nutrition is properly absorbed, immunity remains balanced, and waste is efficiently eliminated. When Agni is weak or irregular, even good food produces poor results. A simple example is two people eating the same diet—one remains energetic while the other gains weight or feels tired. Ayurveda explains this difference through the quality of Agni, not through calories alone. Modern science now recognizes this as metabolic efficiency and mitochondrial function.

Ayurveda also described the body as a **tissue hierarchy** through the concept of **Dhatu**. According to this model, nourishment flows sequentially from one tissue to the next—blood nourishes muscle, muscle nourishes fat, fat supports bone, bone supports marrow and nerves, and so on. If digestion is poor at the beginning, all tissues downstream suffer. This explains why chronic digestive problems can eventually lead to anemia, weak muscles, joint problems, hormonal imbalance, and low immunity. Modern medicine observes the same pattern but often treats each tissue problem separately rather than correcting the source.

The concept of **Srotas**, or channels, further highlights Ayurveda's systems thinking. Srotas include not only blood vessels and lymphatics but also microscopic transport and communication pathways that deliver nutrients, remove waste, and transmit signals. When these channels are clear, tissues receive proper nourishment and toxins are removed efficiently. When they are blocked—due to inflammation, metabolic waste, or poor circulation—disease begins. For example, blocked coronary arteries cause heart disease, blocked lymphatic flow causes swelling, and blocked neural communication causes sensory or motor dysfunction. Ayurveda described these processes long before modern imaging techniques existed.

Another unique aspect of the Ayurvedic blueprint is **Kala**, the recognition that time and rhythm are essential to health. The body is designed to function according to daily, seasonal, and life-stage cycles. Digestion, hormone release, sleep, immunity, and mental clarity all follow predictable rhythms. Ayurveda emphasized daily routines (Dinacharya) and seasonal adaptations (Ritucharya) to maintain harmony with these cycles. A simple example is sleep—staying awake late at night disrupts digestion, hormones, and immunity. Modern science now explains this through circadian rhythm disruption and hormonal imbalance, confirming the ancient insight.

The strength of Ayurveda lies in its ability to **connect structure, function, timing, and regulation into a single blueprint**. While modern science uses terms such as homeostasis, feedback loops, tissue signaling, and biological clocks, Ayurveda used Dosha, Agni, Dhatu, Srotas, and Kala to describe the same reality. The language is different, but the principles are strikingly similar. Both systems recognize that disease arises when regulation fails, communication breaks down, and rhythms are ignored.

This convergence is not accidental. It reflects a shared understanding of the body as an intelligently designed system rather than a collection of isolated parts. Ayurveda's blueprint-based approach allows early detection of imbalance, individualized treatment, and long-term prevention. By focusing on regulation rather than replacement, Ayurveda aims to restore the body's natural self-healing capacity. In this way, Ayurveda represents not an alternative to modern science, but an early and comprehensive form of systems medicine—one that modern healthcare is only now beginning to rediscover.

2.5 Disease as Deviation From the Blueprint

When viewed through the lens of design and engineering, disease is not an enemy attacking the body from outside, but a **warning signal** arising from within. Just as a machine produces noise, heat, vibration, or warning lights when it is overloaded or poorly maintained, the human body produces symptoms when it is forced to function outside its design limits. Pain, fatigue, fever, indigestion, anxiety, and disturbed sleep are not mistakes of the body; they are messages indicating that something in the system is not working as intended. Ignoring these messages does not solve the problem—it allows the damage to deepen.

Ayurveda explained this deviation from normal functioning through clear and practical concepts. **Dosha imbalance** represents disturbed regulation, similar to a control system gone off balance. **Agni dysfunction** means faulty metabolism, where food and experiences are not properly processed. **Ama accumulation** refers to sticky, harmful metabolic residue that clogs tissues and interferes with communication. **Srotas blockage** means impaired transport of nutrients, oxygen, and waste. Modern science describes the same processes using different language—metabolic dysregulation, chronic inflammation, oxidative stress, and failure of cellular signaling. Though the terms differ, both systems describe the same breakdown of order within the body.

A simple example can be seen in chronic indigestion. Occasional indigestion is a warning that food intake, timing, or stress levels are unsuitable. If this signal is ignored and repeatedly suppressed with medication, digestion becomes weaker over time. Undigested food leads to bloating, acidity, and eventually nutrient deficiency. Later, this may progress into obesity, diabetes, or inflammatory disease. Ayurveda describes this as weak Agni and Ama formation, while modern science calls it impaired metabolism and gut inflammation. In both cases, the disease began as a deviation from the digestive blueprint.

Another clear example is chronic stress. The human body is designed to handle short periods of stress followed by recovery. When stress becomes constant—due to work pressure, poor sleep, emotional strain, or digital overload—the nervous and hormonal systems remain in a continuous alert state. High blood pressure, anxiety, insomnia, and weakened immunity appear. Ayurveda describes this as aggravated Vata and Pitta with Ojas depletion. Modern medicine describes it as sympathetic overactivity, cortisol excess, and immune suppression. The disease is not random; it is the predictable result of exceeding the body's stress-handling capacity.

Joint pain and stiffness provide another illustration. The body is designed for balanced movement and proper load distribution. Poor posture, lack of exercise, excess weight, and repeated strain disturb this balance. Early stiffness and mild pain are warning signs. If ignored or suppressed, cartilage slowly wears away, leading to osteoarthritis. Ayurveda explains this through Vata imbalance, tissue dryness, and poor nourishment of Dhatus. Modern science explains it through mechanical overload, inflammation, and reduced cartilage repair. In both views, the disease is a signal that the movement blueprint has been violated.

Even lifestyle diseases such as diabetes and heart disease follow this pattern. The body is not designed for constant overeating, refined foods, irregular sleep, and inactivity. Initially, the body compensates by increasing insulin production or raising blood pressure to maintain circulation. These compensations keep the system functioning temporarily. Over time, however, compensation becomes failure. Ayurveda calls this prolonged Dosha disturbance and Agni exhaustion; modern medicine calls it insulin resistance and vascular disease. The disease is not sudden—it is the final stage of long-term deviation.

Both Ayurveda and modern science agree on a critical principle: **treating symptoms without correcting the underlying deviation ensures recurrence**. Lowering blood sugar without correcting diet, sleep, and stress does not restore metabolic intelligence. Reducing pain without correcting movement patterns does not restore joint health. Suppressing inflammation without removing its cause allows deeper damage to continue silently. This is similar to repeatedly resetting an alarm without fixing the problem that triggered it.

True health engineering, therefore, begins much earlier. It asks fundamental design-based questions: What is the human body designed to eat? How much physical and mental load can it safely handle? How much rest does it require? What rhythms must be respected? Which early signals must never be ignored? Ayurveda answered these questions through individualized lifestyle guidance, seasonal routines, and preventive care. Modern science now validates these principles through systems biology and preventive medicine.

When disease is understood as a deviation rather than an enemy, the approach to health changes completely. The goal shifts from fighting disease to **restoring alignment with the body's blueprint**. By correcting inputs, reducing overload, clearing metabolic waste, and supporting natural repair mechanisms, the body often heals itself. In this way, disease becomes not a failure of the body, but a reminder to return to the design rules that sustain health.

2.6 The Human Body as a Self-Designed Intelligent System

All machines created by humans depend completely on external intelligence. A car needs engineers to design it, workers to assemble it, drivers to operate it, and mechanics to repair it. Even the most advanced computers and robots require programmers, regular updates, an external energy supply, and scheduled maintenance. If left unattended, machines slowly deteriorate and eventually stop working. The human body is fundamentally different. It is the only known system that **designs itself, builds itself, operates itself, repairs itself, and adapts continuously**, all without external supervision. This makes the human body not just a biological structure, but a self-designed intelligent system.

This self-design begins at the very first moment of life. From a single fertilized cell, the body creates trillions of specialized cells—nerve cells, muscle cells, blood cells, skin cells—each with a specific role. These cells do not randomly appear; they follow precise instructions, communicate with one another, and arrange themselves into tissues and organs in the correct place and sequence. For example, the heart forms early and starts beating before the brain is fully developed, ensuring circulation for the growing body. No engineer stands inside the womb directing this process. It unfolds automatically through internal intelligence. No factory on Earth can take raw material and produce a fully functioning, conscious human being.

A simple everyday comparison helps clarify this uniqueness. If a house is being built, masons, electricians, plumbers, architects, and supervisors are all required. If a mistake occurs, external correction is needed. In contrast, the human body builds itself inside the womb without any conscious control. If minor errors occur at the cellular level, many are corrected automatically, or the faulty cells are eliminated. This ability to self-correct during construction is unmatched by any man-made system and reflects deep biological intelligence.

The body's intelligence does not stop after birth. Throughout life, it continuously **repairs itself**. Skin heals after cuts, bones mend after fractures, blood cells are replaced every few months, and the liver can regenerate even after part of it is removed. These repairs occur without conscious effort or external command. A machine with a broken wire or cracked part cannot repair itself; it waits for a technician. The human body, however, detects damage, mobilizes resources, and restores function from within. When this repair ability weakens—as in diabetes, aging, or severe stress—healing becomes slow, showing that disease is often a failure of repair intelligence rather than just damage.

The human body also **adapts continuously** to changing conditions. Muscles grow stronger with regular use, lungs adapt to high altitude by increasing oxygen-carrying capacity, and immunity becomes stronger after exposure to infections. Even the brain changes its structure with learning, a phenomenon known as neuroplasticity. This means the body not only survives stress but can become better because of it—within limits. Machines do not grow stronger by being used; they wear out. The human body, when used intelligently, becomes more efficient and resilient.

Another unique feature of the human body is its ability to **learn from experience**. The immune system remembers past infections, allowing a faster response in the future. Metabolism adapts to dietary patterns, and the nervous system refines movements and skills through practice. For example, learning to ride a bicycle feels difficult initially, but once learned, it becomes automatic. This learning is stored not in a single location but across multiple systems. Ayurveda recognized this long ago through the concept of Samskara—impressions formed by repeated experiences that shape future responses.

Most importantly, the human body possesses **self-awareness**, something no machine has. Humans experience pain, pleasure, emotion, memory, intention, and reflection. This awareness allows conscious decision-making, ethical judgment, and self-observation. A machine can process data, but it does not know that it is processing. The presence of awareness allows humans to participate actively in their own healing—by changing habits, managing stress, and understanding bodily signals.

Ayurveda explained this self-designed intelligence through the science of **Garbha Sharira**, which describes how the body forms and develops under the influence of **Beeja** (the genetic seed), **Dosha** (functional regulation), **Agni** (transformative intelligence), and **Kala** (time and sequence). These principles ensured that development followed a precise order—just as modern embryology shows that organs form in a fixed sequence governed by genetic signals and chemical gradients. Today, science explains this using terms such as gene expression, cellular signaling, and morphogen gradients, confirming the same underlying truth.

Understanding the human body as a self-designed intelligent system changes how we view health and disease. Disease is not simply a mechanical failure; it is often a sign that the body's intelligence is overloaded, confused, or deprived of proper conditions. Supporting health, therefore, means supporting this intelligence—through proper nutrition, rest, movement, emotional balance, and timely care. When the body's natural design is respected, healing becomes smoother, recovery becomes faster, and long-term health becomes achievable.

2.7 Self-Repair and Regeneration

One of the most remarkable differences between the human body and any machine is the ability to repair itself continuously. Machines wear out with use. Metal fatigues, parts loosen, wiring degrades, and once damage occurs, an external technician is required to fix it. In contrast, the human body is designed with **built-in repair mechanisms** that operate day and night without conscious control. Skin renews itself every few weeks, blood cells are replaced regularly, the lining of the gut regenerates within days, bones heal after fractures, and even the liver can regrow lost tissue. These processes show that repair is not an emergency response—it is a constant background function of life.

At the microscopic level, this repair intelligence becomes even more impressive. Every day, our cells are exposed to damage from normal metabolism, environmental toxins, radiation, and stress. Yet the body is equipped with **DNA repair enzymes** that correct genetic damage thousands of times daily. Without this continuous correction, life would not be possible even for a short period. Similarly, the immune system constantly identifies and removes damaged, aged, or abnormal cells before they can become harmful. Cancer does not occur because abnormal cells appear—such cells arise daily—but because repair and surveillance systems fail to eliminate them in time. This highlights that health depends more on **repair efficiency** than on the absence of damage.

A simple everyday example helps make this clear. When you accidentally cut your finger, you do not need to instruct the skin on how to heal. Bleeding stops, a clot forms, new tissue grows, and the skin closes on its own. This same intelligence repairs muscles after exercise, strengthens bones after load-bearing activity, and restores tissues after illness. Machines cannot improve themselves through use, but the human body becomes stronger when stressed within limits. Exercise strengthens muscles and bones, exposure to mild infections strengthens immunity, and learning strengthens neural connections. This ability to grow through repair is unique to living systems.

Aging is often misunderstood as an inevitable breakdown. In reality, aging represents a **gradual decline in regenerative intelligence**, not sudden failure. In youth, repair is fast and efficient—wounds heal quickly, infections resolve easily, and energy returns rapidly. With advancing age, repair becomes slower due to reduced stem cell activity, mitochondrial inefficiency, hormonal changes, and cumulative stress. The body still repairs itself, but with less precision and reserve. This explains why older individuals take longer to recover from illness or injury. Aging, therefore, is not merely the passage of time, but the gradual weakening of self-repair systems.

Ayurveda recognized this truth thousands of years ago and developed **Rasayana**, the science of rejuvenation, to preserve and strengthen the body's repair intelligence. Rasayana is not simply a treatment for disease; it is a method of maintaining the quality of repair throughout life. Classical texts describe Rasayana as that which stabilizes aging, promotes longevity, strength, immunity, memory, and intellect. In simple terms, Rasayana aims to keep the body "younger" by maintaining its ability to repair damage efficiently and correctly.

A practical example of Rasayana can be seen in recovery after illness. Two people may suffer from the same infection and receive similar treatment. One recovers quickly with restored strength, while the other remains weak and fatigued for months. Ayurveda explains this difference through the quality of Ojas and Rasayana support—the internal reserve that determines how well repair occurs. Modern science explains the same difference through immune resilience, mitochondrial recovery, and stem cell support. Both perspectives point to the same conclusion: **healing speed depends on repair intelligence, not just treatment.**

Rasayana also plays an important role in mental and nervous system repair. Stress, poor sleep, and emotional strain damage neural circuits over time. Without proper restoration, this leads to anxiety, depression, poor memory, and reduced concentration. Ayurveda emphasized that Rasayana nourishes not only the body but also the mind, preserving clarity and stability. Modern research now confirms that neuro-regeneration, synaptic repair, and mitochondrial health are essential for mental well-being—exactly what Rasayana aims to protect.

From a modern scientific viewpoint, Rasayana supports key repair systems such as **stem cell function, mitochondrial energy production, immune balance, and neuroplasticity**. For common man perspective, it keeps the body's "repair workshop" well-stocked, well-powered, and well-coordinated. Without this support, the body still repairs itself, but slowly and imperfectly, leading to chronic illness and premature aging.

Understanding self-repair and regeneration changes how we view health. Disease is not always the result of damage alone; it is often the result of **failed or inadequate repair**. Supporting the body's natural repair mechanisms—through proper nutrition, rest, stress management, movement, and rejuvenative practices—is therefore more important than fighting disease aggressively. When repair intelligence is strong, the body can overcome many challenges naturally. In this sense, true medicine does not replace broken parts—it restores the wisdom that knows how to repair them.

2.8 Adaptation: The Core of Health

Machines are designed to function best under fixed conditions. If temperature, load, fuel quality, or operating speed changes too much, machines begin to malfunction or break down. Living systems are fundamentally different.

The human body survives and thrives not by resisting change, but by **adapting to it**. Every day, the body adjusts to variations in physical activity, climate, food availability, emotional experiences, and exposure to germs. This ability to adjust continuously is the true foundation of health.

Modern science explains this adaptive ability through the concepts of **plasticity** and **allostasis**. Plasticity means the body's structures and functions can change in response to experience. Allostasis means the body maintains stability not by staying the same, but by changing appropriately. For example, when you exercise regularly, muscles become stronger, bones denser, and the heart more efficient. These changes are not signs of stress or damage; they are healthy adaptations. Ayurveda described this same intelligence through **Dosha dynamics**, especially the role of **Vata**, which governs movement, communication, and responsiveness throughout the body.

A simple example of healthy adaptation is seen in people who move to a high-altitude area. Initially, they may feel breathless or tired because oxygen levels are low. Over time, the body adapts by producing more red blood cells to carry oxygen efficiently. Once adaptation is complete, the person can function normally again. This process occurs automatically. If adaptation fails, altitude sickness develops. This illustrates that symptoms are not enemies, but signs that adaptation is still in progress or has been exceeded.

Adaptation also explains how the body responds to physical stress, such as exercise. When muscles are used beyond their usual level, tiny injuries occur. The body responds by repairing these fibers and making them stronger. If exercise is done regularly with proper rest, strength and endurance increase. If the load is excessive or recovery is inadequate, pain, inflammation, or injury develops. Ayurveda explains this as balanced or aggravated Vata, while modern science describes it as an appropriate or excessive stress response. In both views, health depends on **matching load with recovery capacity**.

Nutrition provides another clear example of adaptation. The body can handle occasional overeating or fasting because it is designed with flexible metabolic pathways. However, constant overnutrition, irregular eating, or poor-quality food overwhelms these adaptive mechanisms. Initially, the body compensates by increasing insulin or storing excess energy as fat. Over time, this adaptation becomes maladaptive, leading to obesity, diabetes, and metabolic syndrome. Ayurveda describes this as disturbed Agni and Kapha accumulation; modern science calls it metabolic overload and insulin resistance. The disease emerges only when adaptation limits are crossed.

Psychological and emotional adaptation is equally important. The human body is designed to handle short-term stress, such as danger or challenge, followed by recovery. In modern life, stress often becomes continuous—due to work pressure, emotional strain, poor sleep, and constant stimulation. The nervous system remains in a constant alert state. Initially, this increases performance, but eventually it leads to anxiety, high blood pressure, digestive problems, and weakened immunity. Ayurveda describes this as aggravated Vata and Pitta; modern science describes it as chronic sympathetic activation and cortisol excess. In both systems, disease appears when **stress exceeds adaptive capacity**.

Sleep plays a central role in restoring adaptation. During sleep, the body repairs tissues, resets hormones, clears brain waste, and strengthens immunity. Occasional sleep loss can be tolerated, but chronic sleep deprivation overwhelms adaptive systems. Memory declines, immunity weakens, and emotional balance is lost. Ayurveda emphasized proper daily rhythm (*Dinacharya*), while modern science highlights circadian biology. Both agree that ignoring biological timing damages adaptive balance.

Health, therefore, is not about maintaining perfect, unchanging conditions. It is about maintaining **adaptive balance**—the ability to respond to challenges and return to stability. Ayurveda called this state *Samatva*, meaning balanced functioning despite constant change. When adaptation is respected, the body becomes resilient. When adaptation is ignored or overloaded, disease develops gradually.

Understanding adaptation shifts the focus of healthcare. Instead of fighting symptoms, we learn to ask: Is the body being overloaded? Is recovery adequate? Are rhythms respected? Are stressors appropriate for the individual's capacity? By supporting adaptation—through proper nutrition, movement, rest, emotional regulation, and lifestyle alignment—we strengthen the body's natural ability to stay healthy. In this sense, adaptation is not just a feature of life; it is the **core definition of health itself**.

2.9 Learning and Biological Memory

Learning is commonly associated with the brain—studying, remembering facts, or acquiring skills. However, modern biology has revealed that **learning occurs throughout the entire body**, not just in the mind. Muscles, immune cells, metabolic systems, and even genes adjust their behavior based on past experiences. This ability to remember and adapt improves efficiency and survival. At the same time, when unhealthy patterns are repeated, the body "learns" disease. In simple terms, the body becomes good at whatever it practices—whether health or illness.

A clear example of biological learning is seen in muscles. When a person begins exercising, movements initially feel difficult and tiring. With repeated practice, muscles grow stronger, and movements become easier. This happens because muscle fibers and nerve connections adapt to repeated use. However, the opposite is also true. Prolonged inactivity teaches the body to conserve muscle, leading to weakness and stiffness. The body has learned a pattern—either strength or decline—based on repeated behavior. This shows that learning is not just mental; it is deeply physical.

The immune system also demonstrates powerful biological memory. When the body encounters a germ for the first time, it takes time to fight it. After recovery, the immune system remembers that germ and responds faster if it appears again. This learning protects us from repeated infections and forms the basis of vaccination. However, immune learning can also go wrong. In allergies, the immune system repeatedly misinterprets harmless substances—such as pollen or food—as dangerous. Over time, this mistaken response becomes stronger. Ayurveda described this as faulty Samskara in the immune response, while modern science calls it immune sensitization. In both cases, the system has learned the wrong lesson.

Metabolism provides another simple illustration of biological memory. If a person repeatedly consumes excess sugar and calories, the body adapts by producing more insulin to manage the load. Over time, cells become less responsive to insulin. This condition, known as insulin resistance, is not a sudden failure—it is the result of long-term metabolic learning. Even when the diet improves, the body may continue to behave as if overload is present, because the pattern has been deeply learned. Ayurveda explained this through repeated Agni disturbance and Ama formation, highlighting that disease becomes habitual if the pattern is not consciously corrected.

Stress and emotional experiences also leave lasting impressions on the body. Repeated exposure to stress trains the nervous system to remain in a constant alert state. This leads to anxiety, sleep disturbance, digestive problems, and high blood pressure. The danger may no longer be present, but the body continues to react as if it is. Modern science describes this as stress conditioning and altered neural circuits. Ayurveda described the same phenomenon through **Samskara**—mental and physical impressions stored from repeated experiences. This explains why simply removing stressors may not immediately restore calm; the body has learned a pattern of overreaction.

Even at the genetic level, experiences leave marks. Modern research shows that diet, stress, toxins, and lifestyle can influence gene expression through epigenetic changes. These changes do not alter the genes themselves but modify how strongly certain genes are switched on or off. This means the body remembers past experiences at a molecular level. Ayurveda anticipated this idea by recognizing that long-standing habits shape constitution and disease tendency. Health, therefore, reflects not just current behavior but the accumulated memory of past choices.

Because disease is often learned, **healing must involve re-learning**. Suppressing symptoms without changing underlying patterns is like correcting handwriting errors without teaching the correct letters. Ayurveda emphasized **Abhyasa**—repeated practice of healthy habits—to overwrite unhealthy Samskaras. Regular sleep, mindful eating, proper movement, breath regulation, and mental discipline gradually teach the body a new pattern. Modern rehabilitation, behavioral therapy, and lifestyle medicine follow the same principle, though described in different terms.

Understanding biological learning transforms the approach to treatment. Disease is not merely something to be removed; it is something that has been practiced over time. To heal deeply, the body must be guided to **unlearn disease patterns and relearn balance**. When healthy signals are repeated consistently, the body's memory shifts. In this way, true healing is not an instant correction, but a process of intelligent re-education—aligning the body's learned behavior back with its original blueprint.

2.10 Self-Awareness: The Ultimate Differentiator

The greatest difference between a human being and any machine lies not in speed, strength, or intelligence, but in **self-awareness**. Machines can collect information, analyze patterns, and even learn through programming, but they do not experience what they do. A computer can detect damage; it does not feel pain. A robot can recognize emotions; it does not experience fear, joy, or compassion. Humans, on the other hand, live with continuous inner experience. We feel hunger, pain, happiness, sadness, fatigue, motivation, and meaning. This ability to experience and reflect on experience is what makes human life unique.

Modern science recognizes consciousness as an emergent property of complex brain activity, but Ayurveda described this long before neuroscience existed. According to Ayurveda, life exists through the integration of **Sharira** (the physical body), **Manas** (the mind that thinks and feels), and **Atma** (the principle of awareness or witnessing). When these three function in harmony, health is complete. If the body is healthy but the mind is disturbed, suffering remains. If the body and mind function, but awareness is clouded, decisions become harmful. This is why Ayurveda never separated physical health from mental clarity and self-awareness.

A simple everyday example shows the importance of self-awareness in health. Two people may have the same physical condition, such as mild back pain. One person listens to the body's signals, rests appropriately, corrects posture, and recovers quickly. The other ignores pain, continues overexertion, suppresses symptoms with medication, and eventually develops chronic back problems. The difference is not strength or treatment, but awareness.

Self-awareness allows early recognition of imbalance and timely correction, preventing disease progression.

Self-awareness also plays a powerful role in emotional health. Humans can observe their own thoughts and emotions. A person may notice anger rising, reflect on its cause, and choose not to act impulsively. This ability to observe rather than react is absent in machines. When awareness is weak, emotions control behavior, leading to stress-related illness, addictions, and destructive habits. When awareness is strong, individuals can change their responses, reducing stress and supporting healing. Ayurveda recognized that mental clarity directly influences physical balance, while modern science confirms that emotional regulation affects hormones, immunity, and nervous system function.

Chronic pain provides another clear example. Pain is not just a physical signal; it is deeply influenced by attention, emotion, and meaning. Two people with similar injuries may experience very different levels of pain depending on fear, anxiety, or calmness. Modern research shows that mindfulness and awareness-based therapies can reduce pain perception even without changing the injury itself. This does not mean pain is imaginary—it means awareness modifies how the body processes signals. Ayurveda understood this by emphasizing the role of Manas and Atma in the experience of suffering.

Self-awareness also enables **intentional healing**, something machines cannot perform. A person can consciously choose to improve sleep, reduce harmful habits, manage stress, or seek support. These choices are guided by awareness of long-term consequences, not immediate impulses. Machines follow instructions; humans can change them. This ability makes lifestyle-based healing possible. Without awareness, even the best medical advice fails because habits remain unchanged.

Yoga was developed as a practical science to strengthen and stabilize self-awareness. Yoga does not merely stretch muscles or improve breathing; it trains attention and reduces mental noise. Through practices such as posture, breath control, and meditation, the mind becomes calmer and awareness becomes clearer. When mental fluctuations settle, the nervous system relaxes, hormonal balance improves, and immune regulation becomes more stable. Modern studies confirm that yoga improves stress tolerance, emotional regulation, and overall well-being by influencing brain and autonomic function.

Health, therefore, is incomplete without clarity of awareness. A body may be treated, and symptoms may be controlled, but if awareness remains clouded, the same harmful patterns return. Ayurveda emphasized that true healing involves recognizing one's own tendencies, limits, and needs. Yoga provides tools to reconnect with this inner intelligence. In this sense, self-awareness is not a philosophical luxury—it is a biological necessity.

The ultimate differentiator between humans and machines is not intelligence alone, but the ability to know that one is alive, to observe oneself, and to choose consciously. This awareness transforms intelligence into wisdom. When awareness guides action, the body's natural regulatory systems function smoothly. When awareness is ignored, even the most advanced medical interventions remain incomplete. True health arises when the body, mind, and awareness work together in harmony.

2.11 Structural Blueprint: Cells, Tissues, and Organs

At the most fundamental level, the human body is built from **cells**, which function like tiny intelligent processors. Each cell generates its own energy, performs specific tasks, communicates with neighboring cells, and repairs itself when damaged. Unlike electronic microprocessors, cells are living units capable of adapting to changing conditions. Inside each cell are **mitochondria**, often called the "power plants" of the body, which produce energy needed for all activities. When mitochondrial function begins to decline, the first symptom is often unexplained fatigue. This is why long-lasting tiredness frequently appears years before a formal diagnosis of disease—it is an early warning that cellular energy production is under strain.

A simple example can be seen in chronic tiredness despite normal medical reports. Blood tests may appear normal, yet the person feels exhausted. This often reflects early cellular energy failure rather than organ disease. If ignored, this energy deficit gradually affects tissues and organs.

Ayurveda recognized this early stage through weakened **Agni** at the tissue level, explaining why restoring digestion and metabolism often improves energy before disease becomes obvious.

Cells do not function in isolation. They organize into **tissues,** which are groups of similar cells working together for a common purpose, much like individual components forming a circuit. Muscle tissue produces movement, bone tissue provides structure, nerve tissue transmits information, and blood tissue transports oxygen and nutrients. For tissues to remain healthy, they require continuous nourishment, adequate oxygen, proper movement, and balanced load. If tissues are underused, overused, or poorly nourished, their function gradually declines. For example, prolonged sitting weakens muscles and reduces circulation, while excessive repetitive strain damages tendons and joints.

Ayurveda describes tissue health through the concept of **Dhatus,** which represent a sequential hierarchy of nourishment. According to this model, nutrients are first processed and then distributed step by step to different tissues. If digestion is poor at the beginning, all tissues suffer later. This explains why long-standing digestive problems can eventually lead to muscle weakness, joint pain, hormonal imbalance, and low immunity. Modern medicine observes these patterns but often treats each tissue problem separately, whereas Ayurveda traces them back to the same source.

Organs represent the highest level of structural organization. Each organ is a specialized machine designed for a specific task—the heart for pumping blood, lungs for gas exchange, liver for metabolism and detoxification, kidneys for filtration, and brain for coordination. Organs are robust and have significant reserve capacity. They rarely fail suddenly without warning. Most organ diseases develop after years of cellular and tissue dysfunction. By the time an organ shows visible damage on scans or tests, the underlying problem has often existed for a long time.

For example, liver disease does not appear overnight. Years of poor diet, alcohol intake, medications, or metabolic stress slowly damage liver cells. The liver compensates for a long time because of its large reserve and regenerative capacity. Symptoms appear only when damage crosses a threshold. Similarly, heart disease develops silently through gradual vessel damage and metabolic imbalance long before chest pain or a heart attack occurs. These examples show that organ failure is the **final stage of a long process**, not the beginning.

Joint disorders provide another clear illustration of the structural hierarchy. Cartilage damage does not start at the joint alone. It often begins with muscle imbalance, poor posture, reduced circulation, and metabolic inflammation at the tissue level. When muscles fail to support joints properly, excessive load reaches cartilage. Over time, this leads to degeneration. Replacing the joint may relieve pain, but if tissue imbalance remains, other joints begin to suffer. Ayurveda explained this through poor nourishment of **Asthi Dhatu** (bone tissue) following disturbance in earlier Dhatus.

Understanding the structural blueprint of cells, tissues, and organs changes how disease is interpreted. Instead of seeing disease as sudden organ failure, it is recognized as a **progressive breakdown starting at the cellular level**. Early symptoms such as fatigue, mild pain, stiffness, or digestive discomfort are not trivial—they are early signs of structural imbalance. Addressing problems at this stage is far easier than repairing organs later.

Ayurveda's Dhatu model aligns closely with modern systems biology. Both emphasize that health depends on proper digestion, efficient energy production, continuous nourishment, and balanced use of tissues. When these foundational processes are maintained, organs function smoothly. When they are neglected, disease becomes inevitable. Respecting this structural hierarchy allows healthcare to move from late-stage repair to early-stage preservation, protecting the body's architecture before irreversible damage occurs.

2.12 Functional Blueprint: Nervous, Endocrine, and Immune Software

Just as a modern machine depends not only on hardware but also on software to function correctly, the human body depends on **functional control systems** that regulate how organs behave. The nervous system, endocrine system, and immune system together act as the body's biological software. Organs may be structurally intact, yet disease can arise when this software becomes disordered. Modern science increasingly recognizes that many chronic illnesses begin as functional disturbances long before any visible organ damage occurs. Ayurveda described the same principle by focusing on regulation, rhythm, and intelligence rather than isolated organs.

The **nervous system** is the body's master control network. It processes information faster than any computer and does so using remarkably little energy. It coordinates movement, sensation, emotions, digestion, heart rate, breathing, and sleep—often without conscious awareness. In daily life, this system is constantly adapting to stress, workload, and environmental demands. When the nervous system is overloaded for long periods, regulation begins to fail. For example, a person under chronic stress may develop poor sleep, digestive upset, anxiety, palpitations, and fatigue, even though all medical tests appear normal. These symptoms reflect nervous system overload rather than organ disease. If this overload continues, it eventually contributes to high blood pressure, diabetes, depression, and heart disease. Ayurveda identified this early stage as Vata imbalance, while modern medicine calls it autonomic dysfunction.

The **endocrine system** works as chemical programming, sending hormonal instructions through the bloodstream. Hormones do not build tissues directly; instead, they decide timing—when to grow, store energy, release energy, rest, or reproduce. When hormonal signals are mistimed or excessive, the body's coordination breaks down. A common example is hypothyroidism, where the thyroid gland may be structurally normal, but hormone output is low. The person experiences weight gain, cold intolerance, sluggish digestion, and fatigue—not because organs are damaged, but because the metabolic software is running slowly. Similarly, conditions like polycystic ovary syndrome (PCOS) occur when hormonal communication between the brain and ovaries is disturbed. Ayurveda interpreted these states as Agni disturbance and Kapha–Vata imbalance, focusing on restoring rhythm rather than replacing organs.

The **immune system** functions as an intelligent defense network rather than a simple attack force. Its job is to recognize danger, respond appropriately, remember past threats, and stand down when the threat is gone. When this intelligence is compromised, disease arises in predictable ways. If immune strength is low, infections occur frequently. If immune discrimination fails, the body attacks its own tissues, leading to autoimmune diseases like rheumatoid arthritis or thyroid disorders. If immune surveillance weakens, abnormal cells escape detection and may develop into cancer. These failures are not random. They reflect loss of balance, clarity, and regulation within the immune system. Ayurveda described this through concepts of Bala (defense strength), Ojas (resilience), and Ama (toxic interference).

Everyday examples make this clear. A person under chronic emotional stress often catches colds repeatedly. The stress hormones suppress immune function, reducing resistance. Another person may develop allergies, where harmless substances trigger exaggerated immune responses. This reflects faulty immune learning and discrimination. In older adults or chronically ill patients, reduced immune surveillance increases cancer risk. In all these cases, the problem is not simply germs or genes—it is failure of immune regulation.

Yoga and Ayurveda address these functional problems at their root. Yoga calms the nervous system through breath regulation, movement, and meditation. This reduces stress hormones, improves sleep, and restores autonomic balance. Ayurveda supports endocrine health by strengthening Agni, respecting daily and seasonal rhythms, and correcting metabolic disturbances. Together, they help clear Ama, restore tissue communication, and enhance immune intelligence. For example, regular yoga practice often improves blood pressure, blood sugar, and anxiety without directly targeting organs. Similarly, Ayurvedic dietary and lifestyle measures can normalize hormonal cycles and reduce autoimmune flare-ups by restoring systemic balance.

Understanding the functional blueprint changes how health and disease are viewed. Disease is not always a broken part; often, it is a **misinformed or overloaded control system**. Treating only organs without correcting nervous stress, hormonal rhythm, and immune clarity is like repairing machinery while ignoring faulty software. True healing begins by restoring regulation. When the nervous system becomes calm, hormones regain rhythm, and the immune system regains discrimination, the body's natural intelligence takes over. In this way, Yoga and Ayurveda do not fight disease directly; they restore the software that allows the body to heal itself.

2.13 Energy Blueprint: Fuel, Conversion, and Distribution

Every system that functions—whether a car, a factory, or a living body—depends first on **energy**. No machine fails only because of broken parts; most failures begin with wrong fuel, inefficient energy conversion, or ignored warning signs. The human body follows the same rule. Health depends not merely on how much energy we consume, but on **what type of fuel we use, how efficiently it is converted, and how well it is distributed to every cell**. Ayurveda recognized this fundamental law thousands of years ago and built its entire health science around food compatibility, digestive intelligence, and respect for biological timing.

Food is the primary fuel of the human body, but food is more than calories. It carries chemical instructions that influence hormones, immunity, and metabolism. Two meals with the same calorie count can have very different effects on energy. For example, a meal of fresh, simple, well-cooked food provides steady energy and mental clarity. In contrast, ultra-processed food high in sugar, refined flour, and unhealthy fats may give a quick burst of energy followed by fatigue, heaviness, and irritability. Modern science explains this through blood sugar spikes and inflammation. Ayurveda described the same phenomenon by distinguishing between compatible food (Ahara) that nourishes tissues and incompatible food that creates Ama—sticky metabolic residue that blocks energy flow.

Digestion and conversion of fuel are more important than the amount consumed. A person may eat nutritious food, yet feel tired, bloated, or heavy if digestion is weak. This is similar to a good engine running poorly because combustion is inefficient. In the body, digestion is governed by Agni—the metabolic intelligence that transforms food into usable energy. When Agni is balanced, food becomes energy, warmth, and tissue nourishment. When Agni is weak or irregular, food remains partially digested, producing toxins and fatigue. This explains why people with indigestion, acidity, or irregular eating habits often feel low energy even with adequate nutrition.

Oxygen is the second essential component of energy production. Just as fire needs oxygen to burn fuel, cells need oxygen to convert nutrients into ATP—the body's energy currency. Poor breathing habits, anemia, lung disease, or a sedentary lifestyle reduce oxygen delivery. This results in early fatigue, brain fog, and poor endurance. Ayurveda and Yoga emphasized **Prana**, the life force carried by breath, as central to energy health. Simple practices like slow breathing, walking, and posture correction improve oxygen utilization and energy efficiency, often relieving fatigue without medication.

Sunlight and biological rhythm play a critical role in energy regulation. Modern science shows that sunlight exposure regulates circadian rhythms, influencing sleep, hormone release, digestion, and energy use. When people stay indoors, work late nights, or sleep irregularly, energy systems fall out of sync. They may experience poor sleep, low morning energy, weight gain, and mood disturbances. Ayurveda emphasized Kala—the influence of time—and prescribed daily routines (Dinacharya) to align the body with natural rhythms. Ignoring biological time is like running a machine continuously without maintenance—it eventually overheats and fails.

Sleep is the body's primary energy restoration phase. During deep sleep, tissues repair, hormones reset, and energy reserves are replenished. Chronic sleep deprivation disrupts energy distribution, leading to tiredness, irritability, poor immunity, and metabolic disease. A person may rely on stimulants like caffeine to push through fatigue, but this only masks the problem. Ayurveda viewed sleep as one of the three pillars of health and warned that poor sleep drains Ojas, the body's reserve of vitality.

When **wrong fuel is repeatedly used, digestion is ignored, and warning signs are suppressed**, metabolic toxicity builds silently. Early signals include heaviness after meals, sluggishness, gas, poor appetite, mood changes, and sleep disturbance. These are not minor complaints; they are dashboard warnings. If ignored, they progress into obesity, diabetes, fatty liver disease, and cardiovascular problems. Modern medicine often detects disease only when lab values become abnormal, but Ayurveda emphasizes correcting the imbalance at the symptom stage itself.

Understanding the energy blueprint allows for prevention instead of late repair. Choosing compatible food, eating at regular times, supporting digestion, breathing well, getting sunlight, and respecting sleep cycles keeps energy systems clean and efficient. When energy flows smoothly, tissues are nourished, organs perform effortlessly, and the mind remains clear. Disease arises not because the body is weak, but because its energy rules have been violated for too long.

In essence, **energy health is the foundation of all health**. The human body is remarkably forgiving, but not limitless. By understanding fuel, conversion, and distribution—and by honoring the principles described by Ayurveda and confirmed by modern science—health can be preserved long before disease demands repair.

2.14 Conclusion: Engineer Health, Don't Chase Disease

The human body is not a passive machine—it is a self-designed, adaptive, learning, and self-aware system. Treating such a system without understanding its blueprint is the greatest engineering mistake in medicine. Understanding the blueprint transforms healthcare from crisis repair into preventive engineering, from symptom suppression into intelligence restoration.

- Machines obey intelligence.
- The human body embodies intelligence.
- Respecting this truth is the future of medicine.

Chapter 3

Preventive Engineering: Why Most Diseases Are Man-made

3.1 Introduction – Disease is Not An Accident

In engineering science, failure never happens suddenly. A bridge collapses only after years of corrosion, overloading, inferior material quality, and neglected maintenance. Long before the final collapse, there are visible cracks, rust, vibrations, and warning signs that are repeatedly ignored. Machines break down in the same manner—not because of a single bad day, but due to continuous misuse, wrong inputs, lack of servicing, and disregard of early alerts. The human body follows exactly the same principles of biological engineering. Disease is therefore rarely an accident or a stroke of bad luck. In most cases, it is the final outcome of long-term errors related to diet, stress, sleep, posture, emotions, addictions, and daily habits.

From a common man's perspective, people often say, "I suddenly got diabetes," or "The heart attack came without warning." In reality, the warning signs were present for years—weight gain, fatigue, acidity, disturbed sleep, breathlessness, anxiety, or joint stiffness—but were considered normal or ignored. Just as a vehicle gives warning through reduced mileage, unusual sounds, or overheating, the body gives subtle signals long before disease becomes visible on reports or scans. Disease is not a sudden enemy; it is a slow message from the body that has been neglected for a long time.

Modern medicine has achieved extraordinary success in emergency care and organ repair. Heart surgeries, insulin therapy, dialysis, ventilators, and intensive care units save millions of lives. However, modern medical systems are largely reactive. They intervene after structural damage has already occurred. For example, blood pressure medicines are started after hypertension is diagnosed, insulin is given after diabetes is established, and joint replacement is advised after cartilage is destroyed. While these interventions are lifesaving, they address the consequence rather than the cause.

Preventive medicine—and Ayurveda in particular—works at a fundamentally different level. Instead of waiting for a breakdown, it focuses on designing health so that failure never arises. Ayurveda clearly states that a person who regularly follows wholesome food (*hitāhāra*), proper daily routine (*vihāra*), and balanced use of body and mind remains free from disease. This principle is not philosophical or spiritual alone; it is deeply practical and based on centuries of systematic observation of cause and effect.

3.1.1 Clinical Example 1: Type 2 Diabetes

From a clinical standpoint, type 2 diabetes is often diagnosed when fasting and post-meal blood sugar levels are high. However, research clearly shows that insulin resistance begins 10–15 years before diagnosis. During this long, silent phase, patients commonly experience abdominal obesity, tiredness, post-meal sleepiness, increased hunger, and stress intolerance. These are not "normal signs of aging" but early metabolic alarms. Ayurveda recognizes this stage as a weakening of *Agni* (metabolic fire). If corrected early with dietary regulation, physical activity, stress management, and routine discipline, diabetes can often be prevented entirely.

Example

A person continuously eats late-night dinners, consumes sugary tea multiple times a day, avoids physical activity, and sleeps poorly due to stress. For years, nothing dramatic happens. Gradually, weight increases, energy decreases, and digestion becomes sluggish. Eventually, a blood test labels the condition as diabetes. The disease did not arrive suddenly; it was patiently constructed by daily habits.

3.1.2 Clinical Example 2: Heart Disease

Heart attacks are often perceived as sudden, catastrophic events. Clinically, however, atherosclerosis (plaque buildup in arteries) starts in early adulthood. Years of a high-fat diet, smoking, mental stress, lack of sleep, and a sedentary lifestyle cause silent inflammation and narrowing of blood vessels. Symptoms such as chest heaviness on exertion, breathlessness, acidity-like pain, or fatigue are early warning signs. Ayurveda correlates this with *Rasavaha* and *Raktavaha Srotas* dysfunction, meaning impaired circulation and nourishment of tissues.

Example

Just as a water pipe gets blocked slowly by internal deposits before water flow suddenly stops, arteries also narrow gradually before a heart attack occurs. The final event looks sudden, but the process is old.

3.1.3 Clinical Example 3: Osteoarthritis

Knee osteoarthritis is commonly diagnosed when X-rays show joint space narrowing. However, cartilage degeneration begins many years earlier due to obesity, faulty posture, lack of muscle strength, repetitive joint strain, and inflammation. Early signs such as morning stiffness, mild pain after walking, or cracking sounds are often ignored. Ayurveda describes this gradual tissue depletion as *Dhatu kshaya*. Early intervention with weight control, movement correction, and nourishment can delay or prevent severe joint damage.

3.1.4 Engineering Insight Applied to Medicine

In engineering, preventive maintenance is cheaper, safer, and more effective than emergency repair. The same principle applies to human health. Treating disease after it appears is like repairing a collapsed bridge—costly, risky, and sometimes incomplete. Preventing disease is like maintaining the bridge regularly so that collapse never occurs.

3.2 The Human Body as a Living Engineering System

The human body is not a random collection of organs but a precisely organized, self-regulating, and adaptive living engineering system. Every structure and function in the body operates under intelligent control networks that constantly sense, analyze, and respond to both internal and external conditions. The nervous system functions like a high-speed real-time control unit, instantly processing sensory information and issuing commands. The endocrine system acts as chemical programming, releasing hormones that regulate growth, metabolism, reproduction, stress response, and repair over longer time scales. The immune system serves as an intelligent defense, surveillance, and repair network, capable of recognizing threats, remembering past exposures, and distinguishing between self and non-self. Together, these systems continuously maintain internal balance, known scientifically as homeostasis and described in Ayurveda as *Swasthya*—a state of dynamic equilibrium.

From a Common man's perspective, this coordination can be understood by comparing the body to a modern automated factory. Sensors detect changes, computers process information, and automated systems correct errors without human intervention. For example, when body temperature rises, sweating is automatically triggered; when blood sugar increases, insulin is released; when an infection enters, immune cells are activated. None of these requires conscious effort. Disease occurs when these intelligent systems are repeatedly overruled, overloaded, or deprived of proper support.

3.2.1 Essential Conditions for Optimal Functioning

Like any engineered system, the human body requires certain fundamental conditions to perform optimally. The first requirement is correct inputs. Nutritious food provides raw materials and energy, clean air supplies oxygen for cellular respiration, water maintains biochemical reactions, sunlight regulates biological clocks and vitamin D synthesis, and positive sensory impressions support mental stability. Clinically, poor inputs lead to predictable outcomes. For instance, diets high in refined sugar and processed foods result in insulin resistance and metabolic syndrome, while lack of sunlight contributes to vitamin D deficiency, bone weakness, and immune dysfunction.

A simple example is is fuel quality in a vehicle. Even the most advanced car will malfunction if filled with contaminated or low-grade fuel. Similarly, the body cannot function properly when fed junk food, polluted air, or constant negative sensory input such as noise, screens, and emotional stress.

3.2.2 Load Regulation: Respecting Biological Capacity

The second requirement is proper load regulation. Every system has a design limit. Physical activity strengthens muscles and joints when within capacity, but excessive or repetitive strain causes injury and degeneration. Mental work improves cognition when balanced, but chronic mental overload leads to anxiety, burnout, and hormonal imbalance. Emotional stress, when brief, enhances survival responses, but when prolonged, damages the cardiovascular, metabolic, and immune systems.

Clinically, prolonged sitting leads to back pain, obesity, and insulin resistance. Chronic workplace stress contributes to hypertension, depression, and heart disease. Ayurveda describes this state as *Ati-yoga*—excessive utilization beyond adaptive capacity. A layman's analogy is overloading an electric circuit. Initially, the system heats up; if the overload continues, fuses blow or wiring burns. The body behaves similarly when biological limits are ignored.

3.2.3 Regular Maintenance: Daily Servicing of the Body

The third requirement is regular maintenance. In engineering, machines require lubrication, cooling, cleaning, and scheduled servicing. In the human body, maintenance is achieved through sleep, rest, proper digestion, and regular elimination of waste. Sleep allows neural repair, hormonal recalibration, and immune restoration. Digestion converts food into usable energy and tissues, while elimination removes metabolic waste.

Clinically, chronic sleep deprivation is associated with obesity, diabetes, depression, and immune suppression. Constipation, acidity, and bloating indicate failure of digestive maintenance. Ayurveda emphasizes *Dinacharya* (daily routine) and *Ritucharya* (seasonal routine) to ensure regular servicing of the body. Everyone can relate this to skipping oil changes in a vehicle—initially, the car runs, but internal damage accumulates silently.

3.2.4 Timely Repair and Recovery Mechanisms

The fourth requirement is timely repair. The body possesses a remarkable self-healing capacity, but this requires adequate recovery time. Minor tissue injuries, infections, and metabolic imbalances can be fully repaired if the body is allowed to rest and recover. Detoxification processes in the liver, kidneys, gut, and skin continuously neutralize and eliminate harmful substances.

Clinically, repeated infections, delayed wound healing, and chronic fatigue indicate failure of repair mechanisms. Ayurveda uses interventions like *Panchakarma* to support detoxification and tissue rejuvenation before irreversible damage occurs. A layman's analogy is repairing small cracks in a wall before they become structural failures.

3.2.5 Disease as Network Failure: Systems Biology Perspective

Modern systems biology strongly supports this engineering view of the body. Disease is now understood not as a problem of a single organ, but as a failure of interconnected networks. For example, diabetes is not merely a pancreatic disorder but involves muscle, liver, fat tissue, brain, and immune signaling. Heart disease is not just a cardiac problem but involves metabolic, inflammatory, hormonal, and psychological factors.

When one system is chronically overloaded or neglected, imbalance spreads across networks. Poor sleep disrupts hormonal balance, which affects metabolism, immunity, and mental health. Chronic gut dysfunction alters immune regulation, leading to systemic inflammation and autoimmune tendencies. Ayurveda described this interconnected spread centuries ago through the concept of *Srotas* (body channels) and *Dosha* imbalance.

3.3 Disease Development – Stages of Failure (Shat-Kriya-Kala)

3.3.1 The Myth of "Sudden Disease"

A common belief among patients is that diseases like diabetes, blood pressure, heart disease, or arthritis appear suddenly. People often say, "I was perfectly fine until last month." This belief is dangerous because it prevents people from recognizing early warning signs. Scientific reality strongly contradicts this idea. No chronic disease develops overnight. What appears sudden is only the diagnosis, not the disease itself.

Both modern medicine and Ayurveda confirm that disease develops silently, gradually, and predictably, often over many years. Symptoms are not the beginning of disease; they are late alarms indicating that the body's compensatory capacity has been exhausted. By the time pain, abnormal blood reports, or organ damage appear, the disease process is already well established.

3.3.2 Disease as a Gradual Engineering Failure

To understand this easily, consider a machine. Initially, efficiency drops slightly. Fuel consumption increases, noise develops, and performance reduces. If these signs are ignored, parts begin to wear out. Eventually, the machine breaks down completely. The human body behaves in the same way. Early symptoms such as fatigue, acidity, constipation, mild joint stiffness, or disturbed sleep are not minor problems; they are warning signals of internal imbalance.

3.3.3 Clinical Example: Type 2 Diabetes Mellitus

Type 2 diabetes is an excellent example of slow biological failure. In the first three years, insulin resistance develops silently. Body cells stop responding properly to insulin, yet blood sugar levels may remain normal. There are no obvious symptoms, but internally, excess sugar intake, lack of physical activity, chronic stress, and fat accumulation begin to disturb metabolism.

Between years four and six, early functional disturbances appear. A person may feel tired easily, gain weight around the abdomen, feel hungry frequently, or become sleepy after meals. Modern medicine calls this early metabolic syndrome. Ayurveda describes this phase as weakening of *Agni*, the digestive and metabolic fire, meaning the body can no longer process nutrients efficiently.

After few years and ten, prediabetes develops. Blood sugar levels become borderline, HbA1c rises mildly, and symptoms like increased thirst and urination may appear. Ayurveda calls this stage *Prasara*, where imbalance spreads from its original site into the whole system. Finally, after sometimes, diabetes is diagnosed when blood sugar remains persistently high, and medication becomes necessary. The key insight is that the diagnosis is new, but the disease process is often 10–15 years old.

3.3.4 Explanation According To Ayurveda: Shat-Kriya-Kala

Ayurveda explains disease development in six stages known as *Shat-Kriya-Kala*. These stages range from early accumulation of imbalance (*Sanchaya*) to full manifestation (*Vyakti*) and complications (*Bheda*). Modern medicine usually detects disease only in the later stages, when symptoms and lab abnormalities are obvious. Ayurveda aims to intervene much earlier, when correction is simple, reversible, and cost-effective.

3.3.5 Additional Clinical Example: Knee Osteoarthritis

Knee osteoarthritis also follows a slow failure pattern. In early years, a person experiences mild morning stiffness or discomfort after prolonged sitting. In the middle stage, pain appears after walking or climbing stairs. In late stages, severe pain occurs along with X-ray changes. Importantly, cartilage degeneration begins many years before severe pain is felt. By the time radiological damage is visible, the disease has already progressed significantly.

3.3.6 Why the Myth of Sudden Disease Is Harmful

Believing that a disease is sudden causes people to ignore early warning signs. The preventive window is missed, the disease becomes chronic, and lifelong treatment becomes necessary. Early intervention during simple symptoms like fatigue, mild weight gain, acidity, constipation, or stress can prevent or even reverse many chronic diseases.

3.4 Man-Made Disease – Poor Fuel (Dietary Errors)

In engineering science, the quality of fuel directly determines the performance, efficiency, and lifespan of an engine. Even a well-designed machine fails prematurely when repeatedly supplied with contaminated or unsuitable fuel. The human body follows the same biological engineering rule. Food is not merely a source of calories; it is the primary raw material for cellular energy, tissue repair, hormonal balance, and immune strength. When nutrition quality is poor, metabolic systems are forced to operate under abnormal conditions, leading to gradual dysfunction and disease.

From a clinical standpoint, poor dietary habits are now recognized as the leading cause of non-communicable diseases worldwide. Refined sugar causes repeated spikes in blood glucose and insulin, eventually leading to insulin resistance and type 2 diabetes. Trans fats and repeatedly heated oils damage the inner lining of blood vessels (endothelium), accelerating atherosclerosis and increasing the risk of heart attacks and strokes. Ultra-processed foods—rich in preservatives, artificial colors, emulsifiers, and refined carbohydrates—disturb gut microbiome, increase intestinal permeability, and trigger chronic low-grade inflammation. This inflammatory state is now known to be a common underlying factor in obesity, diabetes, cardiovascular disease, autoimmune disorders, and certain cancers.

3.4.1 Fuel Quality and Engine Life

A simple example is adulterated petrol or diesel. Initially, the vehicle may run without obvious trouble, but mileage drops, engine noise increases, and overheating becomes frequent. Over time, injectors clog, cylinders wear out, and the engine fails prematurely. Similarly, the human body may appear normal for years despite poor eating habits. Gradually, signs such as weight gain, acidity, bloating, fatigue, skin problems, and disturbed sleep appear. These are early indicators that the "fuel" is damaging the system.

3.4.2 Refined Sugar and Diabetes

Clinically, excessive consumption of refined sugar—found in sweets, soft drinks, packaged juices, bakery items, and even hidden in sauces—leads to repeated insulin overload. Over time, body cells become resistant to insulin, forcing the pancreas to work harder. Eventually, insulin production declines and diabetes manifests. Ayurveda describes this process as weakening of *Agni* and accumulation of *Ama* (metabolic toxins), which block metabolic pathways.

An example is continuously revving an engine at high speed. Initially, performance seems strong, but internal components wear out faster, leading to breakdown.

3.4.3 Trans Fats and Heart Disease

Trans fats, commonly present in bakery products, fried snacks, margarine, and fast food, are particularly harmful. They increase bad cholesterol (LDL), reduce good cholesterol (HDL), and promote inflammation within blood vessels. Clinically, this results in early plaque formation, hypertension, and coronary artery disease. Ayurveda warns against stale, reheated, and incompatible foods (*Viruddha Ahara*), which disturb tissue nutrition and circulation.

For example this is like pourring thick sludge into narrow pipes. Flow reduces gradually until blockage occurs.

3.4.4 Ultra-Processed Foods and Gut Damage

Ultra-processed foods lack natural fiber and are rich in chemical additives. Scientific research shows that these foods disrupt gut bacteria, leading to dysbiosis. The gut, which plays a central role in immunity and metabolism, becomes inflamed and leaky. Clinically, this manifests as bloating, acidity, irritable bowel syndrome, allergies, autoimmune diseases, and even mood disorders due to the gut-brain connection.

Ayurveda recognized the importance of digestion thousands of years ago, stating that even nutritious food acts like poison if not properly digested. The concept of *Ahara Vidhi* (rules of eating) emphasizes freshness, proper combination, and mindful eating.

3.4.5 Processed vs Fresh Food

A fresh home-cooked meal nourishes the body much like clean fuel runs an engine smoothly. Packaged food is like processed industrial fuel—convenient but damaging when used regularly. Occasional consumption may not cause immediate harm, but daily dependence creates long-term damage.

3.4.6 Food Compatibility and Timing

Ayurveda places special emphasis on food compatibility and timing. Incompatible food combinations, such as fruit with dairy or heavy meals late at night, overload digestion and produce toxins. Clinically, late-night eating is associated with obesity, reflux disease, fatty liver, and insulin resistance. Modern chronobiology now confirms that eating against the body's biological clock disrupts metabolic regulation.

Example is refueling a machine when it is switched off or overheated—fuel efficiency drops and damage increases.

Preventive Engineering Insight

Most dietary diseases are man-made because they result from repeated wrong choices rather than unavoidable circumstances. Poor fuel does not cause immediate failure; it causes slow degradation. By choosing natural, fresh, seasonal, and well-digested food, the metabolic system remains efficient and resilient. Prevention begins not in hospitals, but in the kitchen.

3.5 Overloading Beyond Biological Design Capacity

Every engineered system is designed to operate within specific load-bearing limits. When these limits are exceeded repeatedly or for prolonged periods, the system initially adapts but eventually fails. The human body follows the same fundamental engineering principle. Physical tissues, metabolic pathways, hormonal systems, and neural circuits all have finite adaptive capacities. Continuous physical, mental, or emotional overload pushes these systems beyond their design limits, resulting in gradual breakdown and disease.

From a biological standpoint, the body is remarkably adaptable. Muscles strengthen with exercise, the brain becomes sharper with learning, and stress hormones help manage short-term challenges. However, when load becomes chronic and recovery is inadequate, adaptation turns into exhaustion. Ayurveda describes this state as *Ati-yoga*, meaning excessive or improper use of body, senses, or mind. Unlike acute stress or exertion, which can be beneficial, chronic overload steadily erodes physiological resilience.

3.5.1 Physical Overload: Structural Breakdown

Physical overload occurs when the body is subjected to repetitive strain, prolonged immobility, or excessive exertion without adequate recovery. Prolonged sitting, a common feature of modern life, leads to weakening of postural muscles, reduced joint lubrication, impaired circulation, and metabolic slowdown. Clinically, this manifests as neck pain, back pain, knee degeneration, obesity, and insulin resistance.

On the other extreme, excessive physical activity without rest—such as overtraining in athletes or heavy labor without recovery—leads to muscle tears, stress fractures, joint degeneration, and chronic fatigue. Ayurveda correlates such conditions with *Vata* aggravation, resulting in pain, stiffness, and degeneration.

Basic Understanding Example:
Just as continuously overloading a bridge with heavy trucks weakens its structure over time, continuously overloading joints or keeping the body immobile for hours weakens muscles and cartilage, eventually causing pain and damage.

3.5.2 Mental Overload: Cognitive and Emotional Exhaustion

Mental overload results from prolonged cognitive demands, multitasking, constant screen exposure, and information overload. The brain is designed for focused work interspersed with rest. Continuous mental strain without pauses leads to reduced concentration, memory problems, irritability, and sleep disturbances.

Clinically, mental overload contributes to anxiety disorders, depression, burnout syndrome, and psychosomatic illnesses. Ayurveda refers to improper use of the mind as *Asatmya Indriyartha Samyoga*, where the senses and mind are overstimulated beyond their natural capacity.

Basic Understanding Example:
A computer running too many applications simultaneously slows down and overheats. Similarly, the human mind becomes inefficient and unstable when overloaded with continuous mental tasks and emotional pressures.

3.5.3 Emotional Overload and Chronic Stress

Emotional overload is one of the most damaging forms of biological stress. Persistent worry, fear, anger, or grief keeps the stress response continuously activated. This disrupts the hypothalamic-pituitary-adrenal (HPA) axis, leading to sustained cortisol release. Over time, this causes hormonal imbalance, immune suppression, increased blood sugar, abdominal obesity, hypertension, and sleep disorders.

Clinically, chronic stress is strongly linked to cardiovascular disease, diabetes, autoimmune disorders, and accelerated aging. Ayurveda recognizes this as *Pragyaparadha*, misuse of intellect, where unhealthy emotional patterns are repeatedly reinforced.

Basic Understanding Example:
It is like keeping a machine running at full speed all the time. Initially, performance seems high, but internal components wear out rapidly, leading to sudden failure.

3.5.4 Sleep Deprivation: Failure of Recovery Systems

Sleep is the primary recovery mechanism of the human body. During sleep, tissues repair, hormones balance, memory consolidates, and immune surveillance is restored. Chronic sleep deprivation deprives the body of its natural repair time.

Clinically, inadequate sleep is associated with obesity, insulin resistance, hypertension, weakened immunity, mood disorders, and impaired cognitive function. Ayurveda considers night sleep essential for *Dhatu poshana* (tissue nourishment) and *Ojas* (vital immunity).

Basic Understanding Example:
Skipping sleep is like skipping maintenance of a factory. Production may continue for some time, but machinery degrades silently until a major breakdown occurs.

3.5.5 Combined Overload: The Modern Lifestyle Trap

Modern lifestyles often combine physical inactivity, mental overwork, emotional stress, and sleep deprivation simultaneously. This multiplies the damage. A person may sit for long hours, face constant work pressure, eat irregularly, sleep late, and repeat the cycle daily. Clinically, this pattern leads to lifestyle disorders such as diabetes, hypertension, obesity, irritable bowel syndrome, infertility, and autoimmune diseases.

Ayurveda warns that imbalance does not remain localized. Overloaded systems disturb others, leading to systemic disease.

3.5.6 Preventive Engineering Perspective

Overload is not harmful by itself; unrelieved overload is. Respecting biological design capacity through balanced activity, scheduled rest, emotional regulation, and adequate sleep preserves system integrity. Periodic unloading through relaxation, exercise, meditation, and routine discipline restores adaptive capacity.

3.6 Lack of Servicing – Failure of Daily Maintenance

In engineering, even the most advanced machines fail if routine servicing is neglected. Engines require regular oil changes, filters must be cleaned, moving parts need lubrication, and worn components must be identified early. Skipping maintenance does not cause immediate failure, but it silently accelerates wear and tear. The human body follows the same biological engineering rule. It is a self-repairing system, but this repair depends entirely on daily maintenance practices. When sleep, regular meals, proper elimination, relaxation, and natural movement are neglected, the body's built-in repair mechanisms gradually fail, leading to chronic disease.

From a biological perspective, daily maintenance allows the nervous, endocrine, immune, and metabolic systems to reset and recover. Sleep recalibrates hormones and repairs tissues. Regular meals synchronize digestion and metabolism. Proper elimination removes metabolic waste. Relaxation reduces stress load. Movement maintains circulation and joint health. Ayurveda collectively describes these practices under *Dinacharya* (daily routine) and *Ritucharya* (seasonal routine), emphasizing that health is preserved not by occasional treatment but by consistent daily care.

3.6.1 Sleep: The Primary Servicing Mechanism

Sleep is the most critical daily servicing process of the human body. During deep sleep, growth hormone is released, damaged tissues are repaired, memory is consolidated, and immune surveillance is strengthened. Clinically, chronic sleep deprivation is associated with obesity, diabetes, hypertension, depression, weakened immunity, and accelerated aging.

Ayurveda states that proper night sleep (*Nidra*) nourishes tissues (*Dhatu*), stabilizes the mind, and maintains vitality (*Ojas*). When sleep is irregular or insufficient, repair remains incomplete.

> **Basic Understanding Example:**
> Skipping sleep is like running a factory without shutting it down for cleaning and maintenance. Production continues initially, but internal machinery wears out rapidly.

3.6.2 Regular Meals and Digestive Rhythm

The digestive system operates optimally on rhythm and regularity. Irregular meal timing, skipping breakfast, late-night eating, or overeating disrupt digestive enzymes, gut hormones, and metabolic signaling. Clinically, this leads to acidity, bloating, constipation, fatty liver, insulin resistance, and nutritional deficiencies.

Ayurveda emphasizes eating at the right time, in the right quantity, and according to digestive strength (*Agni*). Irregular eating produces *Ama* (toxic metabolic residue), which gradually blocks bodily channels and initiates disease.

> **Basic Understanding Example:**
> Eating irregularly is like feeding fuel to a machine at random times—sometimes too much, sometimes too little—causing inefficiency and breakdown.

3.6.3 Elimination: Waste Removal as Preventive Care

Proper elimination of urine, stool, sweat, and metabolic waste is essential for maintaining internal cleanliness. Suppression of natural urges, dehydration, sedentary habits, and poor diet impair elimination. Clinically, this results in constipation, urinary infections, headaches, skin disorders, and systemic inflammation.

Ayurveda considers regular elimination (*Malapravritti*) a sign of health. Accumulated waste creates internal toxicity, weakening digestion and immunity.

> **Basic Understanding Example:**
> Blocked drains in a house eventually cause foul smell, overflow, and structural damage. Similarly, blocked elimination pathways poison the body from within.

3.6.4 Relaxation and Mental Reset

Continuous mental activity without relaxation overloads the nervous system. Relaxation practices such as meditation, deep breathing, leisure activities, and quiet reflection allow the brain to reset. Clinically, lack of relaxation contributes to anxiety, hypertension, irritable bowel syndrome, and sleep disorders.

Ayurveda and Yoga emphasize calming the mind to preserve balance between body and consciousness. Mental rest is as important as physical rest.

> **Basic Understanding Example:**
> A mobile phone needs to be switched off or restarted occasionally to function properly. The human mind also requires periodic shutdowns and resets.

3.6.5 Movement: Daily Lubrication of the Body

Regular natural movement keeps joints lubricated, muscles toned, circulation active, and metabolism efficient. Lack of movement leads to stiffness, muscle wasting, poor circulation, and joint degeneration. Clinically, a sedentary lifestyle is a major risk factor for obesity, diabetes, osteoporosis, and cardiovascular disease.

Ayurveda recommends daily exercise (*Vyayama*) appropriate to one's strength and season. Excessive exercise is harmful, but complete inactivity is equally damaging.

> **Basic Understanding Example:**
> Unused machinery rusts faster than machinery used regularly. Similarly, joints and muscles degenerate when movement is absent.

3.6.6 Seasonal Maintenance: Ritucharya

Just as machines are adjusted for changing environmental conditions, the human body requires seasonal adaptation. Cold, heat, humidity, and daylight variations affect digestion, immunity, and mental state. Ayurveda's *Ritucharya* provides guidelines for diet and lifestyle according to seasons to prevent seasonal illnesses and chronic imbalance.

Clinically, ignoring seasonal adaptation contributes to allergies, respiratory infections, skin disorders, and metabolic fluctuations.

Preventive Engineering Insight

Daily maintenance is not optional; it is mandatory for long-term system stability. Disease often results not from one major mistake, but from thousands of small, neglected routines. Dinacharya and Ritucharya represent preventive engineering manuals for the human body, ensuring that wear and tear is repaired before it accumulates into disease.

3.7 Ignoring Early Warning Signals

In any engineered system, warning signals appear long before complete failure occurs. A rise in engine temperature, a blinking oil light, or unusual noise alerts the operator that corrective action is needed. Ignoring these signals or merely silencing the alarm does not solve the problem; it accelerates damage. The human body functions in exactly the same way. Symptoms are not enemies to be suppressed but adaptive warning signals generated by the body's intelligent control systems to indicate imbalance or overload.

From a biological perspective, symptoms represent the body's attempt to protect itself and restore balance. Pain limits movement to prevent further injury. Fatigue forces rest when energy reserves are depleted. Fever enhances the immune response. Ayurveda recognized this wisdom centuries ago, describing symptoms as expressions of *Dosha* imbalance rather than isolated problems. Suppressing symptoms without correcting the underlying cause is equivalent to disabling a car's dashboard warning lights while continuing to drive.

3.7.1 Gastrointestinal Warning Signals

Constipation, bloating, acidity, and irregular bowel habits are among the earliest and most commonly ignored warning signals. Clinically, constipation reflects impaired gut motility, dehydration, inadequate fiber intake, or nervous system imbalance. Chronic acidity indicates mucosal irritation, excess acid secretion, or poor digestive coordination. If ignored or repeatedly suppressed with laxatives and antacids, these conditions progress to irritable bowel syndrome, ulcers, hemorrhoids, or metabolic disorders.

Ayurveda considers proper digestion and elimination central to health. Disturbed *Agni* produces *Ama* (toxic metabolic residue), which spreads throughout the body and initiates systemic disease.

> **Example:** A kitchen sink that drains slowly is an early sign of blockage. Pouring chemicals may give temporary relief, but unless the pipe is cleaned, complete blockage is inevitable.

3.7.2 Fatigue: The Most Ignored Alarm

Fatigue is often normalized in modern society. People commonly say, "Everyone feels tired." Clinically, persistent fatigue reflects mitochondrial stress, hormonal imbalance, anemia, nutritional deficiency, chronic inflammation, or sleep deprivation. When fatigue is ignored and compensated for with caffeine or stimulants, the underlying energy crisis worsens.

Ayurveda views fatigue as depletion of *Ojas* and imbalance of *Vata*. Early correction through rest, nourishment, and routine prevents progression to chronic fatigue syndrome, depression, or metabolic disease.

> **Example:** Running a battery-powered device until the battery is completely drained repeatedly shortens battery life permanently.

3.7.3 Pain and Stiffness: Mechanical Alarms

Pain and stiffness serve as mechanical warning signals. Joint pain indicates overload, inflammation, or degeneration. Muscle stiffness suggests poor circulation or accumulation of metabolic waste. Clinically, ignoring these signals and continuing the same activities leads to chronic arthritis, disc prolapse, or repetitive strain injuries.

Ayurveda associates pain primarily with *Vata* aggravation and tissue depletion. Early interventions such as rest, correction of posture, lubrication (*Snehan*), and movement therapy prevent irreversible structural damage.

> **Example:** A door that creaks is asking for oil. Ignoring the sound leads to rusted hinges and broken hardware.

3.7.4 Mental and Emotional Warning Signals

Anxiety, irritability, low mood, and sleep disturbance are early neuroendocrine warning signals. Clinically, these symptoms reflect an imbalance in stress hormones, neurotransmitters, and circadian rhythm. If suppressed with sedatives or ignored, they progress to depression, panic disorders, hypertension, and autoimmune diseases.

Ayurveda describes this as an imbalance of *Rajas* and *Tamas* affecting the mind (*Manas*). Yoga and lifestyle correction restore balance before disease manifests.

> **Basic Understanding Example:**
> Ignoring repeated error messages on a computer eventually leads to a system crash.

3.7.5 Skin and Immune Signals

Recurrent infections, allergies, acne, and skin rashes are immune warning signals. Clinically, they suggest chronic inflammation, gut dysbiosis, or immune dysregulation. Suppressing these symptoms with repeated antibiotics or steroids without correcting diet and lifestyle weakens immune intelligence further.

Ayurveda considers the skin a mirror of internal health. Early immune signals indicate internal imbalance rather than external infection alone.

> **Basic Understanding Example:**
> Smoke is a warning of fire. Eliminating smoke without extinguishing the fire worsens damage.

Preventive Engineering Insight

Early warning signals offer a critical window for intervention. At this stage, the disease is functional and reversible. Ignoring or suppressing symptoms converts adaptive responses into structural damage. Preventive medicine focuses on decoding symptoms rather than silencing them.

3.8 Preventive Engineering Through Ayurveda

Preventive engineering in health aims to design a system that avoids failure rather than repeatedly repairing damage. Ayurveda represents one of the world's oldest and most complete preventive health sciences, built precisely on this principle. Instead of focusing only on disease treatment, Ayurveda concentrates on maintaining balance so that disease does not arise. It does this through four foundational pillars: **Ahara (correct nutrition), Vihara (balanced lifestyle), Dinacharya (disciplined daily routine), and Panchakarma (periodic detoxification and reset)**. Together, these pillars function as a comprehensive preventive engineering model for the human body.

Modern medical science increasingly supports this approach. Large population studies show that 70–80% of non-communicable diseases—such as diabetes, heart disease, obesity, hypertension, and many cancers—are preventable through early lifestyle modification. Ayurveda articulated this truth thousands of years ago using practical, individualized, and systems-based principles.

3.8.1 Ahara – Correct Nutrition as Primary Design Input

Ahara is considered the most important pillar because food becomes the body itself. Ayurveda emphasizes not only *what* we eat, but *how*, *when*, and *according to whose digestive capacity*. Correct nutrition supports strong digestion (*Agni*), proper tissue formation (*Dhatu*), and balanced immunity (*Ojas*). Food that is fresh, seasonal, compatible, and eaten in the right quantity maintains metabolic efficiency and prevents toxin formation.

Clinical Example:

Patients with early metabolic syndrome often improve dramatically with dietary correction alone—reducing refined carbohydrates, eating at fixed times, and choosing whole foods. Blood sugar, lipid levels, and inflammation markers improve even before medications are introduced.

Basic Understanding Example:
Just as a building made with quality raw materials lasts longer, a body nourished with proper food remains strong and resilient. Junk food may satisfy hunger temporarily, but it weakens the structure over time.

3.8.2 Vihara – Balanced Lifestyle and Load Management

Vihara refers to daily activities, physical movement, mental behavior, emotional regulation, and interaction with the environment. Ayurveda teaches moderation—neither excess nor deficiency. Balanced physical activity strengthens muscles and joints, while adequate rest preserves energy. Emotional balance prevents chronic stress and hormonal disruption.

Clinical Example:
Patients with hypertension often show significant blood pressure reduction through stress management, regular walking, and sleep correction—sometimes reducing the need for lifelong medication.

Basic Understanding Example:
A machine that runs continuously without rest overheats and breaks down. Similarly, a person who works continuously without relaxation develops stress-related illnesses.

3.8.3 Dinacharya – Disciplined Daily Routine as Maintenance Protocol

Dinacharya provides a structured daily routine aligned with biological rhythms. Waking early, proper elimination, regular meals, appropriate activity, relaxation, and timely sleep synchronize the nervous, endocrine, and digestive systems. This rhythm stabilizes metabolism and immunity.

Clinical Example:
Irregular routines are strongly associated with obesity, acid reflux, irritable bowel syndrome, and sleep disorders. Establishing regular meal and sleep timings often resolves symptoms without heavy medication.

Basic Understanding Example:
Just as machines perform best when operated on a fixed schedule, the human body thrives on routine. Irregular habits confuse internal timing systems and cause breakdown.

3.8.4 Panchakarma – Periodic Detoxification and System Reset

Panchakarma is not merely disease treatment; it is preventive maintenance. Environmental toxins, metabolic waste, stress byproducts, and undigested residues accumulate over time despite good habits. Panchakarma removes these burdens, restores digestive strength, rejuvenates tissues, and resets regulatory systems.

Clinical Example:
Patients undergoing Panchakarma often experience improvement in chronic inflammatory conditions, autoimmune tendencies, digestive disorders, and fatigue by restoring systemic balance before irreversible damage occurs.

Basic Understanding Example:
Just as periodic deep cleaning of machinery improves performance and lifespan, Panchakarma cleans internal systems so the body functions smoothly.

Integration of the Four Pillars

These four pillars are not independent; they work synergistically. Correct food supports lifestyle balance, routine stabilizes digestion and sleep, and detoxification enhances the effectiveness of nutrition and routine. Ignoring even one pillar weakens the entire preventive framework.

Modern preventive medicine now echoes this integrated view, recognizing that lifestyle correction, stress management, diet, and periodic health assessment are more powerful than late-stage treatment.

Preventive Engineering Insight

Ayurveda does not wait for disease labels. It intervenes at the level of imbalance, fatigue, indigestion, stress, and subtle dysfunction—when correction is simple and reversible. This is the essence of preventive engineering: **designing daily life in such a way that disease has no opportunity to arise**.

3.9 Mental Preventive Engineering (Pragyaparadha)

Mental preventive engineering addresses the most subtle yet powerful cause of disease: **wrong decisions made despite knowing what is right**. Ayurveda identifies this fundamental error as **Pragyaparadha**, meaning misuse or failure of intelligence. Unlike ignorance, Pragyaparadha occurs when a person is aware of healthy principles but repeatedly chooses actions that violate them. Over time, these repeated mental errors translate into physical disease. Thus, many chronic illnesses do not begin in the body but in the mind.

From an engineering perspective, Pragyaparadha is comparable to an operator overriding safety protocols despite warning signs. The machine itself may be well-designed, but incorrect operation leads to failure. Similarly, the human body may be genetically sound and structurally normal, yet continuous wrong choices—overeating despite fullness, sleeping late despite fatigue, suppressing emotions, ignoring stress, or indulging in addictions—gradually overload biological systems.

3.10 Mind-Body Feedback Loop: The Control System

The mind and body are linked through continuous two-way feedback involving the nervous system, endocrine hormones, and immune signaling. Thoughts, emotions, and perceptions instantly influence heart rate, blood pressure, digestion, immunity, and metabolism. Chronic mental patterns, therefore, produce predictable physiological changes. Persistent fear increases stress hormones, anger elevates inflammatory mediators, and prolonged grief suppresses immunity.

Modern neuroscience and psychoneuroimmunology confirm this Ayurvedic insight. Chronic mental stress alters hypothalamic-pituitary-adrenal (HPA) axis function, disrupts circadian rhythm, and creates low-grade inflammation—the biological foundation of many non-communicable diseases.

3.10.1 Clinical Example 1: Stress-Related Hypertension

Clinically, many patients with hypertension have no primary structural heart disease. Instead, they exhibit chronic mental stress, emotional suppression, competitive behavior, and poor coping mechanisms. Despite knowing the importance of relaxation, exercise, and sleep, they continue stressful lifestyles. This is Pragyaparadha in action.

Yoga-based interventions—breathing practices, meditation, and relaxation—have been shown to reduce blood pressure by improving autonomic balance and lowering cortisol levels.

> **Basic Understanding Example:**
> Continuously pressing the accelerator even when the engine is overheating eventually causes a breakdown. Stress keeps the body in constant "high-speed mode."

3.10.2 Clinical Example 2: Lifestyle Diseases and Emotional Eating

Many individuals know that excessive sugar, junk food, and late-night eating are harmful, yet continue these habits due to emotional triggers such as anxiety, loneliness, or boredom. Clinically, this leads to obesity, diabetes, fatty liver, and digestive disorders. The root cause is not lack of information but lack of mental regulation.

Ayurveda explains that an uncontrolled mind (*Rajas* and *Tamas* dominance) drives unhealthy sensory indulgence, disturbing digestion and metabolism.

> **Basic Understanding Example:**
> Knowing that a road is damaged yet choosing it repeatedly leads to vehicle damage. Knowledge without application fails to protect health.

3.10.3 Clinical Example 3: Autoimmune and Psychosomatic Disorders

In many autoimmune and psychosomatic conditions, emotional stress precedes physical symptoms. Chronic unresolved conflict, fear, or grief alters immune discrimination, leading to inflammatory or autoimmune responses. Clinically, conditions such as rheumatoid arthritis, psoriasis, irritable bowel syndrome, and migraine often worsen during emotional stress.

Yoga and meditation improve emotional awareness, reduce stress reactivity, and restore immune regulation by calming neural and hormonal pathways.

> **Basic Understanding Example:**
> A thermostat set incorrectly causes continuous overheating or cooling. Emotional imbalance sets the body's internal regulation to a harmful setting.

3.11 Yoga as Mental Preventive Engineering

Yoga is not merely physical exercise; it is a systematic method of mental engineering. Practices such as *Asana*, *Pranayama*, *Dhyana*, and ethical disciplines (*Yama* and *Niyama*) strengthen attention, self-control, and emotional stability. This directly prevents Pragyaparadha by aligning knowledge with behavior.

Clinically, yoga improves heart rate variability, reduces inflammatory markers, enhances sleep quality, and stabilizes mood. These changes represent measurable improvements in mind-body regulation.

Preventive Engineering Insight

Pragyaparadha is the earliest and most correctable stage of disease causation. Correcting thought patterns, emotional responses, and decision-making prevents downstream physical damage. Mental preventive engineering, therefore, offers the highest return on health investment.

3.12 Core Principles of Preventive Engineering

Preventive engineering in health is based on the understanding that the human body is an intelligent, self-regulating system designed to preserve balance and survival. Disease does not arise as punishment, fate, or sudden misfortune. Instead, it is **information**—a message generated by the body to indicate that adaptive limits are being crossed. When this information is understood and acted upon early, disease can be prevented or reversed. When ignored, the same information eventually manifests as structural damage and chronic illness.

From both modern science and Ayurveda, a common principle emerges: **the body always warns before it breaks down**. These warnings appear as subtle functional changes long before the disease is diagnosed. Preventive engineering focuses on decoding and correcting these early signals rather than waiting for advanced pathology.

3.12.1 Disease Is Information, Not Punishment

Disease represents feedback from the biological system. Just as an aircraft warning system alerts pilots to pressure changes or engine strain, symptoms alert individuals to imbalance. Pain signals overload or injury. Fever indicates immune activation. Digestive disturbances reflect metabolic stress.

Viewing disease as punishment leads to fear and suppression; viewing it as information leads to correction and healing.

Clinical Example:
A patient with early fatty liver disease often has mild abdominal discomfort, weight gain, and raised liver enzymes. These findings are not punishments but warnings that diet, alcohol intake, and metabolic load are exceeding liver capacity. Early lifestyle correction can completely reverse fatty liver.

Basic Understanding Example:
A bank balance going negative is not punishment by the bank—it is information that expenses exceed income. Ignoring it leads to debt; correcting it restores stability.

3.12.2 The Body Warns Early and Repeatedly

The human body communicates through multiple layers—physical sensations, emotional changes, energy levels, digestion, and sleep patterns. Early warnings include fatigue, acidity, mild pain, disturbed sleep, irritability, or weight gain. These signals often repeat daily, but because they do not cause immediate disability, they are ignored.

Clinically, chronic diseases such as diabetes, hypertension, and arthritis show long asymptomatic or mildly symptomatic phases. By the time diagnosis is made, the disease process is often many years old. Ayurveda described this progressive warning system through *Shat-Kriya-Kala*, emphasizing early correction.

Example: A crack in a wall appears small at first. Ignoring it allows water seepage, rusting of steel, and eventual collapse. Early repair prevents major damage.

3.12.3 Prevention Is More Effective Than Treatment

Preventive measures act at the functional level, where changes are reversible and inexpensive. Treatment at advanced stages requires medications, surgeries, long-term therapy, and carries the risk of complications. From an economic, clinical, and societal perspective, prevention offers far greater return.

Modern public health data shows that lifestyle modification can prevent the majority of heart disease, diabetes, and stroke. Ayurveda operationalized this principle through daily routine, dietary regulation, seasonal adaptation, and mental discipline.

Clinical Example:
Regular exercise and weight management can reduce the risk of type 2 diabetes by more than 50% in high-risk individuals—far more effective than lifelong medication after disease onset.

Example: Servicing a vehicle regularly costs far less than replacing the engine after a breakdown.

3.12.4 Ayurveda as a True Systems Medicine

Ayurveda does not isolate organs or symptoms. It views the body as an interconnected system involving digestion, circulation, metabolism, immunity, mind, and environment. Disease is understood as a disturbance of system harmony rather than isolated organ failure. This aligns closely with modern systems biology, network medicine, and preventive science.

Modern research now recognizes that inflammation, stress, gut health, sleep, and metabolism interact as networks. Ayurveda recognized these interconnections thousands of years ago through the concepts of *Dosha*, *Dhatu*, *Agni*, and *Srotas*.

Example: Irritable bowel syndrome improves not only with gut-focused therapy, but also with stress management, sleep correction, and dietary modification—demonstrating system-level healing.

Example: Fixing only one leaking pipe does not solve plumbing problems if water pressure and drainage systems are faulty. Ayurveda corrects the entire system.

3.12.5 Shift from Reactive to Proactive Healthcare

Modern healthcare is largely reactive—patients seek help after the disease appears. Preventive engineering shifts focus toward proactive design of daily life to preserve health. This includes educating individuals to recognize early signs, make informed choices, and maintain balance through routine and awareness.

Ayurveda emphasizes that health is an active process requiring daily participation, not a passive state maintained by medicines alone.

Preventive Engineering Insight

Health is maintained not by avoiding hospitals, but by understanding the body's signals and responding intelligently. Disease becomes inevitable only when early information is ignored repeatedly. Prevention transforms healthcare from crisis management into intelligent life design.

3.13 Conclusion – Design a Life Where Disease Cannot Arise

Preventive engineering integrates food, lifestyle, mental discipline, and daily routine to maintain lifelong health. Treating disease is repair. Preventing disease is intelligent design. A well-designed life naturally minimizes the possibility of illness and maximizes health, resilience, and longevity.

Chapter 4

Fuel Engineering: Food as Biological Information

"The quality of fuel determines the life of the machine."

— *Engineering Principle*

4.1 Introduction: Food Is Not Calories, It Is Code

In mechanical engineering, fuel selection is a matter of precision, not convenience. Fuel is chosen to match the exact design, pressure tolerance, temperature range, and combustion characteristics of an engine. A high-compression diesel engine will malfunction if petrol is used, not because petrol is useless, but because it delivers the wrong combustion signal. A jet engine cannot run on crude oil because its combustion dynamics, purity, and burn rate are incompatible. Even small deviations in fuel quality produce knocking sounds, overheating, carbon deposits, reduced efficiency, and finally catastrophic failure. The human body follows the same immutable engineering logic.

However, modern society has dangerously oversimplified food. Food is now discussed mainly in terms of calories, taste, convenience, brand value, and marketing appeal. The most common question asked is, *"How many calories does this contain?"* rather than the far more important question, *"What biological instructions will this food give my body?"* This shift has created a fundamental misunderstanding of nutrition. Calories only measure heat energy, but the human body does not function like a furnace. It functions like a **biological information processor**.

In reality, food is a **biological code**. Every morsel consumed carries chemical signals that directly influence hormone secretion, enzyme activation, gene expression, inflammatory pathways, immune responses, gut microbiota behavior, and brain neurotransmitters. For example, refined sugar sends repeated insulin-spiking instructions, while fiber-rich foods activate satiety hormones and beneficial gut bacteria. Certain fats promote inflammation, while others calm cellular stress. Thus, food does not merely fuel the body—it programs it continuously, moment by moment.

Modern nutritional science, molecular biology, and epigenetics now confirm what Ayurveda clearly stated thousands of years ago. Food has the power to switch genes on or off, amplify or suppress inflammation, accelerate aging, or promote repair. Some foods stimulate fat storage pathways, others enhance energy efficiency. Some calm the nervous system and improve sleep, while others overstimulate stress circuits and disrupt mental balance. Ayurveda summarized this entire concept in one concise statement: **"Ahara Sambhavam Vastu"**—the body is created, maintained, and repaired by food. This means that food is not external to the body; it *becomes* the body.

4.1.1 Clinical Perspective

From a clinical standpoint, this explains why two individuals eating the same number of calories can have entirely different health outcomes. One may develop obesity, diabetes, or inflammation, while the other remains healthy. The difference lies not in calorie count, but in **biological messaging**. Diets high in ultra-processed foods deliver signals that promote insulin resistance, gut dysbiosis, and chronic inflammation, even if total calories appear controlled. Conversely, whole foods rich in natural fibers, micronutrients, and bioactive compounds deliver signals that enhance metabolic flexibility, immune balance, and tissue repair.

For example, two meals of equal calories—one from sugary beverages and refined snacks, the other from whole grains, vegetables, and healthy fats—produce completely different hormonal, inflammatory, and metabolic responses in the body. Clinically, this difference explains why calorie-focused diets often fail while quality-focused dietary interventions succeed.

4.1.2 Layman's Understanding

For a layperson, food can be compared not just to petrol, but to a **software update**. Petrol only keeps the engine running, but software determines *how* the engine runs—smoothly, efficiently, or destructively. A wrong software update can crash even the most advanced computer. Similarly, repeated wrong food signals can crash even a genetically strong and structurally healthy body.

Eating junk food daily is not an act of sudden self-destruction. It is a slow process of uploading faulty instructions—telling the body to store fat, increase inflammation, ignore satiety signals, disturb sleep, and weaken immunity. The body follows instructions faithfully until it can no longer compensate, at which point disease becomes visible.

Preventive Engineering Insight

Understanding food as biological information fundamentally changes the approach to nutrition. Health is not protected by calorie counting alone, but by **information quality**. When food sends correct signals consistently, the body self-regulates, repairs itself, and remains resilient. When food sends wrong signals repeatedly, disease becomes inevitable—even without overeating.

4.2 The Human Digestive System: A Precision Fuel Processing Plant

Unlike machines that burn fuel directly, the human body operates a **multi-stage fuel processing plant** with strict quality control. Food is first **mechanically processed** by chewing, which increases surface area and prepares it for chemical action. Next, **chemical digestion** begins—stomach acid denatures proteins; enzymes from saliva, pancreas, and intestine break carbohydrates, proteins, and fats into absorbable units; bile emulsifies fats for efficient uptake. After digestion, nutrients are **absorbed through the intestinal lining**, transported via blood and lymph, **metabolically converted**, and finally **utilized by cells** to produce ATP—the body's usable energy currency. At each step, regulation and feedback ensure precision; failure at any stage compromises the entire system.

Ayurveda describes this entire cascade with one unifying concept: **Agni**—the digestive and metabolic fire. Agni is not confined to the stomach. It functions at **multiple levels**: (1) digesting food in the gut, (2) transforming nutrients in circulation, and (3) enabling tissue-specific nourishment. When Agni is balanced, food becomes energy, strength, clarity, and immunity. When Agni is weak, irregular, or excessive, **even nutritious food becomes toxic**, forming poorly processed residues that burden tissues.

Modern medicine recognizes these failures as **indigestion, malabsorption, metabolic inefficiency, insulin resistance, chronic inflammation, and mitochondrial dysfunction**. In other words, disease often reflects **processing failure**, not fuel shortage.

4.2.1 Clinical Perspective: Where Processing Fails

Clinically, many patients eat "enough" yet remain fatigued, anemic, bloated, or inflamed. Tests may show normal calorie intake but reveal deficiencies, fatty liver, or insulin resistance. This paradox is explained by **inefficient processing**—poor enzyme activity, altered gut lining, dysbiosis, or impaired mitochondrial ATP generation. For example, patients with chronic gastritis or pancreatic insufficiency may consume adequate protein but fail to absorb amino acids effectively, leading to muscle loss and low immunity.

Ayurveda interprets this as **Agni impairment**. The same meal that nourishes one person may produce heaviness, gas, or lethargy in another—because the **processing plant**, not the fuel, differs.

4.2.2 Understanding: Factory, Not Furnace

A simple way to understand digestion is to imagine a **factory**, not a furnace. Raw materials must be crushed, refined, inspected, assembled, and distributed. If one department malfunctions—say quality control—defective products reach the market. Similarly, if chewing is rushed, enzymes are insufficient, bile flow is poor, or absorption is compromised, the body receives **low-quality outputs**, even from good food.

> **Example:** Eating healthy food with poor digestion is like loading premium fuel into a car with clogged injectors—it sputters, wastes fuel, and damages parts.

4.2.3 Mitochondria: The Final Energy Gate

At the cellular level, mitochondria are the **final combustion chambers** where nutrients are converted into ATP. Chronic stress, inflammation, nutrient deficiencies, and toxin load damage mitochondrial function. Clinically, this appears as persistent fatigue, exercise intolerance, brain fog, and slow recovery—despite "normal" diets. Ayurveda would describe this as downstream Agni failure affecting tissue nourishment.

> **Example:** If a power plant receives coal but its turbines are damaged, electricity output falls. The problem is not coal quantity—it's conversion efficiency.

Engineering Truth Applied to Biology

- **Good fuel + poor tuning** → breakdown (healthy diet with poor digestion still fails)
- **Poor fuel + strong tuning** → temporary survival (robust digestion masks bad habits briefly)
- **Good fuel + optimal tuning** → longevity (right food with strong digestion sustains health)

This explains why young individuals may tolerate junk food temporarily (strong tuning), yet develop disease later when tuning degrades. It also explains why restoring digestion—through meal timing, enzyme support, gut healing, stress reduction, and appropriate routines—often produces rapid clinical improvement.

Preventive Engineering Insight

The primary goal of nutrition is not merely to choose "healthy" foods, but to **optimize the processing plant**. Strengthening digestion, absorption, and cellular conversion ensures that fuel becomes function. Ayurveda's focus on Agni aligns perfectly with modern emphasis on gut health, metabolic flexibility, and mitochondrial integrity.

4.3 Fuel Compatibility: One Diet Does Not Fit All

In engineering, fuel compatibility is non-negotiable. Petrol engines, diesel engines, and hybrid engines are designed with different compression ratios, ignition systems, burn rates, and operating temperatures. Supplying the same fuel to all engines is not equality—it is mechanical negligence. Damage occurs not because the fuel is inherently bad, but because it is **mismatched** to the design. The human body follows the same rule of compatibility.

Similarly, **no single diet suits all human beings**. Each person has a distinct metabolic design shaped by genetics, gut microbiome composition, hormonal balance, stress exposure, age, climate, and activity level.

Ayurveda classified this biological individuality as **Prakriti**—the inborn constitutional pattern that determines how one digests, absorbs, utilizes, and reacts to food. Ignoring individuality leads to predictable patterns of disease, even when the diet is considered "healthy" by general standards.

4.3.1 Why the Same Food Produces Different Outcomes

Clinically, it is common to see two people eating the same diet with opposite results. One person feels energetic, calm, and lean; the other develops bloating, acidity, weight gain, or fatigue. This difference arises because food interacts with **the processor**, not just the plate. Warm, nourishing foods may stabilize one person's digestion while triggering inflammation or heaviness in another. Some individuals gain weight easily with carbohydrates, while others lose weight rapidly under stress and require grounding nourishment.

Ayurveda explains these differences through Prakriti tendencies:

- **Vata-dominant** bodies benefit from warm, moist, nourishing foods and regular meals.
- **Pitta-dominant** bodies require cooling, non-irritating foods to prevent inflammation.
- **Kapha-dominant** bodies thrive on light, dry, stimulating foods and suffer from excess heaviness.

Clinical Example 1: Kapha Mismatch and Metabolic Disease

A Kapha-dominant individual consuming excess dairy, refined carbohydrates, sweets, and cold beverages gradually develops weight gain, insulin resistance, fatty liver, and lethargy. Importantly, dairy or carbohydrates are not universally harmful. In this context, they act as **biologically incompatible fuel**, overloading a metabolism already inclined toward storage and slow turnover. Correcting compatibility—lighter meals, warming spices, timed eating, and regular movement—often reverses early disease without aggressive medication.

Layman's analogy:

Giving diesel to a petrol car does not mean diesel is bad—it means the match is wrong.

Clinical Example 2: Pitta Mismatch and Inflammation

Pitta-dominant individuals often tolerate moderate fats and proteins but react poorly to excessive spicy, fried, acidic, or fermented foods—especially under stress or heat exposure. Clinically, this presents as gastritis, acidity, skin rashes, migraines, or inflammatory bowel symptoms. The same "high-protein" or "spicy" diet that energizes another person becomes inflammatory here. Cooling foods, adequate hydration, and meal timing restore balance by matching fuel to design.

> **Example:** High-octane fuel improves performance in one engine but causes overheating in another.

Clinical Example 3: Vata Mismatch and Degeneration

Vata-dominant individuals often suffer when exposed to cold, dry, raw foods, irregular meals, fasting, or excessive caffeine. Clinically, this leads to bloating, constipation, anxiety, insomnia, joint pain, and weight loss. Diet trends that emphasize raw salads or prolonged fasting may suit others, but aggravate Vata, accelerating degeneration. Warm, cooked, nourishing foods and routine are essential for compatibility.

> **Example:** A lightweight engine designed for city driving fails on constant high-speed highways.

4.3.2 Modern Science Correlates

Modern nutrition science increasingly supports personalization. Differences in **genetic polymorphisms, gut microbiome profiles, insulin sensitivity,** and **stress hormones** explain why standardized diets produce variable outcomes. Precision nutrition and personalized medicine echo Ayurveda's Prakriti concept—confirming that compatibility matters more than universality.

Preventive Engineering Insight

Dietary failure often reflects **mismatch**, not moral failure or lack of discipline. When food matches individual design, digestion improves, inflammation reduces, energy stabilizes, and weight normalizes—often effortlessly. When mismatched, even disciplined eating produces disease over time.

4.4 Food as Hormonal Programming

Modern endocrinology has clearly established that food is one of the strongest regulators of the hormonal system. Hormones are chemical messengers that decide how the body stores energy, burns fuel, repairs tissues, responds to stress, and even how hungry or calm we feel. Every time we eat, we are not just filling the stomach—we are **sending hormonal instructions** to the body.

Refined carbohydrates such as sugar, white flour, sweets, and sugary beverages rapidly increase blood glucose, forcing repeated insulin release. When this happens daily, body cells gradually stop responding to insulin, a condition known as insulin resistance. At the same time, chronic consumption of ultra-processed food disrupts leptin signaling. Leptin is the hormone that tells the brain, *"Enough food, stop eating."* When leptin resistance develops, the brain no longer senses fullness, leading to overeating despite sufficient energy stores. Stress combined with poor diet further elevates cortisol, the primary stress hormone, which promotes abdominal fat storage, muscle breakdown, impaired immunity, and sleep disturbance.

Ayurveda described this entire cascade thousands of years ago using a different but remarkably accurate framework. It stated that **Rasa Dushti** (disturbance in primary nutrition and circulation) gradually leads to **Dhatu Dushti** (damage to tissues such as fat, muscle, bone, and reproductive tissue). This means disease does not begin in organs like the pancreas or liver; it begins in distorted nutritional and hormonal signaling. In modern terms, disease starts as **faulty information flow**, not structural failure.

4.4.1 Clinical Perspective: Hormones Before Disease

Clinically, this explains why laboratory tests may remain "normal" for years while patients experience weight gain, fatigue, mood changes, and cravings. Hormonal imbalance precedes measurable disease. For example, a patient may have normal fasting blood sugar but already suffer from insulin resistance and high insulin levels. Similarly, leptin resistance can exist long before obesity is diagnosed.

Repeated intake of sugar, refined flour, fried food, and sweetened beverages programs cells to store fat, increase inflammatory chemicals, and reduce insulin sensitivity. This process is often misunderstood as overeating or lack of willpower. In reality, it is **wrong hormonal programming delivered daily**, regardless of total calorie intake.

4.4.2 Clinical Example 1: Obesity Without Overeating

Many patients with obesity report that they do not eat excessively. Clinically, their problem is not quantity but **hormonal confusion**. Ultra-processed food disrupts insulin and leptin signaling, making the body store fat even on moderate intake. Correcting food quality often leads to weight loss without strict calorie restriction.

> **Example:** If a thermostat is faulty, the room overheats even when the heater is set low. The problem is the signal, not the heater.

4.4.3 Clinical Example 2: Stress, Cortisol, and Fat Accumulation

In individuals under chronic mental stress, even a moderately unhealthy diet causes disproportionate damage. Elevated cortisol instructs the body to conserve energy, store fat (especially around the abdomen), and suppress immunity. Clinically, such patients develop central obesity, diabetes, hypertension, recurrent infections, and poor wound healing.

Ayurveda recognized this mind–nutrition interaction and warned that disturbed mental states aggravate nutritional imbalance, accelerating tissue damage.

> **Example:** A factory under emergency mode stops maintenance and hoards resources. Stress keeps the body in constant emergency mode.

4.4.4 Clinical Example 3: Muscle Loss and Weak Immunity

High cortisol and insulin resistance not only cause fat gain but also muscle breakdown and immune suppression. Clinically, patients feel weak, tire easily, and suffer frequent infections despite adequate food intake. Ayurveda would describe this as *Dhatu Kshaya*—loss of tissue quality due to faulty nourishment.

4.4.5 Hormonal Programming Starts Early

Hormonal misprogramming begins long before visible disease. Children consuming sugary snacks, packaged foods, and sweetened drinks develop early insulin and leptin resistance. This explains the rise of childhood obesity, early puberty, and adolescent diabetes.

> **Example:** Teaching wrong habits early produces lifelong inefficiency—even if correction is attempted later.

Preventive Engineering Insight

Food acts like a daily instruction manual for hormones. When instructions are correct, the body self-regulates appetite, weight, immunity, and energy effortlessly. When instructions are wrong, no amount of discipline can fully compensate. Correcting hormonal programming through compatible, whole, and timely food is more powerful than treating disease after it appears.

4.5 Incompatible Fuel Combinations (Viruddha Ahara)

Ayurveda made a unique and far-sighted observation: **some foods become harmful when combined**, even though each item may be nutritious on its own. This concept is known as **Viruddha Ahara**—incompatible food combinations. Unlike modern nutrition, which often evaluates foods in isolation (proteins, fats, carbohydrates), Ayurveda evaluated **interaction effects**—how foods behave when eaten together and how they affect digestion, immunity, and tissues over time.

Classic examples include milk with sour fruits, milk with fish, heated honey, fruits taken immediately after heavy meals, or combining foods with opposite digestive requirements. Ayurveda warned that such combinations confuse digestion, produce toxins, and initiate disease gradually—often without immediate symptoms.

4.5.1 Modern Scientific Explanation of Incompatibility

Modern science now explains these effects through several mechanisms. Some combinations cause **protein denaturation** and improper digestion. Others promote **fermentation and gas formation**, altering gut pH and disturbing beneficial bacteria. Certain mixes change the gut microbiome composition, increasing inflammatory species. Over time, repeated immune activation occurs as the gut barrier becomes irritated or “leaky,” allowing partially digested food particles to trigger immune responses.

In simple terms, incompatible foods **overload the digestive system with conflicting instructions**, leading to chronic inflammation rather than efficient nourishment.

4.5.2 Clinical Perspective: Disease Without Deficiency

Clinically, many patients with chronic skin disorders, urticaria, irritable bowel syndrome (IBS), migraines, allergies, and autoimmune conditions do not suffer from lack of nutrients. Instead, they often report long-standing habits of incompatible food intake. Their blood tests may appear normal, yet inflammation persists.

For example, patients consuming milkshakes with sour fruits, yogurt with fruits at night, or frequent seafood-dairy combinations may develop chronic skin rashes or sinus allergies. Eliminating incompatible combinations alone—without adding supplements—often leads to significant symptom improvement.

Clinical insight:

The problem is not *what* they eat, but *how foods are combined.*

4.5.3 Specific Examples Explained Simply

Milk + Sour Fruits:

Milk requires slow digestion and a neutral environment, while sour fruits digest quickly and increase acidity. Together, they cause milk protein curdling in the stomach, leading to fermentation, gas, bloating, skin issues, and mucus formation.

Milk + Fish:

Milk is heavy and cooling; fish is heating and protein-dense. This opposite metabolic signaling confuses digestion and may provoke immune reactions. Clinically, this combination is associated with skin disorders and allergic tendencies.

Heated Honey:

Heating alters honey's natural sugars and enzymes, creating compounds that are difficult to digest. Ayurveda warned that this combination produces toxins. Modern science supports that heating honey changes its chemical profile and increases oxidative stress.

Fruits + Heavy Meals:

Fruits digest quickly. When eaten with or immediately after heavy meals, they get trapped in the stomach, ferment, and produce gas and acidity. This leads to bloating, reflux, and gut discomfort.

Chemistry says some substances are safe. Some substances are safe individually but dangerous when mixed. Similarly, food combinations can change their behavior inside the body.

> **Example:** Mixing bleach and acid creates toxic gas—even though both are commonly used separately. Food works the same way inside the digestive system.

4.5.4 Long-Term Effects of Incompatible Eating

Viruddha Ahara rarely causes immediate illness. Instead, it creates **slow, silent inflammation**. Over the years, this inflammation affects the gut lining, immune tolerance, skin health, joints, and even mental clarity. Ayurveda emphasized that such diseases appear "without clear cause" because the cause is daily, subtle, and ignored.

Modern medicine now recognizes this pattern in conditions like food sensitivities, autoimmune flare-ups, chronic fatigue, and functional gastrointestinal disorders.

Preventive Engineering Insight

From a preventive engineering viewpoint, incompatible food combinations act like **fuel additives that corrode the engine slowly**. The engine keeps running for years, but internal damage accumulates. Avoiding incompatible combinations reduces inflammatory load and allows the body's natural repair mechanisms to function effectively.

Textbook Key Points

- Some foods are harmful only when combined
- Viruddha Ahara confuses digestion and immunity
- Disease may arise despite adequate nutrition
- Gut dysbiosis and inflammation explain many effects
- Avoiding incompatibility is a powerful preventive tool

In summary:

Food quality matters. Quantity matters.
But **compatibility may matter the most**.
Many chronic diseases are not caused by what we eat—but by **what we eat together**.

4.6 Processed Food: Adulterated Fuel

In engineering, adulterated fuel is one of the most dangerous threats to machine longevity. Such fuel may allow the engine to run initially, sometimes even giving a sudden surge of power, but it leaves behind impurities that clog injectors, corrode valves, damage filters, and impair combustion chambers. The engine does not fail immediately; instead, its lifespan shortens silently. **Processed food behaves in exactly the same way inside the human body.**

Processed and ultra-processed foods are designed for shelf life, taste enhancement, and convenience—not for biological compatibility. They often provide rapid energy due to refined sugars and starches, but they lack natural fiber, enzymes, micronutrients, and structural complexity needed for healthy metabolism. At the same time, they introduce chemical additives, emulsifiers, preservatives, artificial colors, and altered fats that the human body did not evolve to process efficiently.

4.6.1 Modern Scientific Perspective: Microscopic Damage

Modern research clearly shows that ultra-processed foods increase **oxidative stress**, damage **mitochondrial function**, disturb **gut microbiota**, and activate chronic low-grade inflammation. Mitochondria—the energy generators of cells—are especially vulnerable. When mitochondrial efficiency declines, cells produce less energy and more toxic byproducts. Clinically, this appears as fatigue, brain fog, poor exercise tolerance, slow healing, and accelerated aging.

Processed food also alters gut bacteria, reducing beneficial species and encouraging inflammatory microbes. Since the gut plays a central role in immunity, hormone regulation, and brain function, this disturbance has widespread effects, contributing to obesity, diabetes, autoimmune diseases, depression, and even cancer risk.

4.6.2 Ayurvedic Explanation: Ama – Metabolic Sludge

Ayurveda described this toxic residue long before modern biochemistry and named it **Ama**. Ama is not just undigested food; it is improperly processed metabolic waste that blocks circulation, weakens digestion, and interferes with tissue intelligence. When Ama accumulates, nutrients fail to reach tissues properly, and waste is not eliminated efficiently. Disease then develops gradually, often without a clear single cause.

In modern terms, Ama corresponds to chronic inflammation, metabolic toxins, oxidized fats, and dysfunctional cellular byproducts.

Clinical Example 1: Fatigue and "Normal Reports"

Clinically, many patients complain of persistent tiredness, body aches, bloating, and poor concentration despite "normal" blood tests. Their diet history often reveals heavy reliance on packaged snacks, sugary beverages, instant foods, and bakery products. The issue is not calorie deficiency but **cellular poisoning**. Reducing processed food intake alone often improves energy and mental clarity within weeks.

Example: The car starts every morning, but mileage keeps dropping and strange noises appear. The problem is fuel quality, not engine size.

Clinical Example 2: Obesity and Inflammation

Ultra-processed foods promote weight gain not just by excess calories, but by altering appetite hormones and promoting fat storage. They are engineered to override satiety signals, leading to continuous eating. Clinically, this results in obesity associated with inflammation, joint pain, insulin resistance, and fatty liver.

Ayurveda would describe this as Ama blocking metabolic pathways and disturbing tissue nourishment.

Clinical Example 3: Children and Early Damage

Children consuming packaged snacks, sugary drinks, and fast food show early signs of insulin resistance, poor immunity, attention issues, and obesity. The damage begins early, long before disease labels appear. This demonstrates that processed food silently programs disease decades in advance.

Processed food is convenient, just like adulterated fuel is cheaper and easily available. Both appear harmless initially. But neither supports long-term performance.

Layman's analogy:

Sludge does not stop an engine immediately—it coats parts slowly, reduces efficiency, and causes early breakdown. Processed food does the same to the human body.

Preventive Engineering Insight

From a preventive engineering perspective, the danger of processed food lies in its **silence**. There is no immediate pain, no instant breakdown. The body compensates for years—until it can no longer do so. By the time the disease is diagnosed, the damage has already accumulated.

Avoiding processed food is not about restriction or fear. It is about **preserving the internal machinery** so that natural repair, immunity, and intelligence remain intact.

4.7 Timing of Fuel Intake: The Forgotten Engineering Rule

In engineering, fuel quality alone does not guarantee safe performance. **The timing of fuel delivery is equally critical.** Supplying fuel when a machine is overheated, overloaded, or shut down reduces efficiency and accelerates wear. The human body follows the same biological engineering principle. Even the *right food*, eaten at the *wrong time*, becomes harmful rather than nourishing.

Ayurveda emphasized this rule thousands of years ago by aligning eating habits with **biological rhythms (Dinacharya)**. It clearly stated that digestive strength (*Agni*) is strongest around midday, moderate in the morning and evening, and weakest at night. Modern chronobiology now confirms this observation through circadian rhythm research, showing that insulin sensitivity, digestive enzyme activity, gut motility, and metabolic efficiency peak earlier in the day and decline as night approaches.

4.7.1 Biological Rhythm and Digestive Capacity

The human body operates on an internal clock regulated by light exposure, hormones, and neural signals. During daylight hours, the body is in an active, metabolically efficient state—designed to digest, absorb, and utilize nutrients. At night, physiology shifts toward repair, detoxification, immune surveillance, and cellular regeneration.

When heavy meals are consumed late at night, digestion competes with repair processes. Food remains undigested longer, leading to acid reflux, bloating, disturbed sleep, and metabolic stress. Over time, this mismatch between food timing and biological rhythm contributes to obesity, insulin resistance, fatty liver disease, and type 2 diabetes.

4.7.2 Clinical Perspective: Disease Without Excess Eating

Clinically, many patients with obesity or diabetes insist they "do not eat much." On closer evaluation, the issue is often **late timing**, not excess quantity. Skipping breakfast, eating irregularly during the day, and consuming large dinners at night force the body to store rather than burn energy.

Late-night eating produces higher blood sugar and insulin responses compared to the same meal eaten earlier. Repeated nightly insulin spikes program the body toward fat storage and metabolic dysfunction.

> **Clinical Example:**
> Two individuals eat identical meals. One eats the main meal at 1 p.m., the other at 10 p.m. Over the years, the late eater develops obesity, reflux, and diabetes, despite similar calorie intake.

4.7.3 Ayurvedic Insight: Agni and Kala (Time)

Ayurveda stressed that food must be compatible not only with constitution (*Prakriti*) but also with **time (*Kala*)**. Midday corresponds to peak digestive fire, making it ideal for the heaviest meal. Evening meals should be lighter, and late-night eating is discouraged because Agni is weak and dominated by restorative processes.

When food is eaten against this rhythm, digestion produces *Ama* (toxic residue), which gradually blocks metabolic pathways.

A simple analogy is refueling a machine.

> **Example:**
> Refueling a generator when it is switched off or overheated does not improve output—it wastes fuel and damages components. Similarly, eating heavy food when the body is in "shutdown and repair mode" leads to waste and damage.

Another example is traffic timing. Driving a heavy vehicle during peak traffic causes congestion and damage, whereas the same vehicle moves smoothly during off-peak hours.

4.7.4 Clinical Example 2: GERD and Sleep Disorders

Patients with gastroesophageal reflux disease (GERD) often have a habit of late dinners followed by immediate sleep. Clinically, correcting meal timing—eating earlier and lighter—often improves symptoms even without long-term medication. This demonstrates that timing alone can correct disease mechanisms.

4.7.5 Clinical Example 3: Shift Workers and Metabolic Disease

Shift workers who eat at night against natural circadian rhythms have a much higher incidence of obesity, diabetes, and cardiovascular disease. This provides strong modern evidence that **timing mismatch**, not food quantity alone, drives disease.

Preventive Engineering Insight

Timing is an invisible but powerful factor in nutrition. The same fuel can nourish or damage depending on when it is supplied. Aligning meals with biological rhythms restores metabolic intelligence without drastic dietary restriction.

Textbook Summary Box

- Digestion follows the circadian rhythm
- Agni is strongest at midday, weakest at night
- Late-night eating promotes fat storage and inflammation
- Disease can occur despite normal calorie intake
- Correct timing restores metabolic efficiency

In summary:

Food eaten at the wrong time becomes metabolic waste.
Health is preserved not only by *what* we eat, but **when** we eat.

4.8 Fuel Quantity: Load vs Capacity

In engineering, every system is designed to operate within a defined **load-bearing capacity**. When load repeatedly exceeds capacity, components overheat, wear accelerates, and failure occurs sooner than expected. The human body follows the same biological engineering rule. **Fuel quantity must match processing capacity**—not appetite, availability, or social habit. Ayurveda expressed this principle succinctly as **Matravat Ahara**—eating in the right quantity according to one's digestive capacity (*Agni*).

Modern medicine confirms that **chronic caloric overload**—even by small daily excess—gradually overwhelms metabolic systems. The pancreas compensates by secreting more insulin; muscles and liver become insulin-resistant; fat tissue expands and becomes inflamed. Over time, this adaptive response turns into **metabolic syndrome**, type 2 diabetes, fatty liver disease, hypertension, and dyslipidemia. Importantly, this progression is slow and silent, which is why it is often underestimated.

4.8.1 Quantity Is Not a Fixed Number—It Is Capacity-Dependent

Ayurveda never prescribed a universal portion size. Instead, it taught that quantity must be adjusted to **individual capacity**, which varies with age, constitution, digestion strength, activity level, season, stress, and illness. A quantity that nourishes a physically active young adult may overload an older, sedentary person. Similarly, the same meal may be tolerated at midday (strong Agni) but cause heaviness and acidity at night (weak Agni).

Clinical insight:

Patients often ask, "How much should I eat?" The correct answer is, "As much as your digestion can process without heaviness, lethargy, or discomfort."

Clinical Example 1: Small Excess, Big Consequences

A common clinical pattern is the patient who "eats normal food" yet steadily gains weight. On careful review, the excess may be only 200–300 calories per day—an extra serving of rice, a late-night snack, or sweetened beverages. Over the years, this small overload forces continuous insulin secretion, leading to insulin resistance and fat accumulation.

Reducing quantity to match capacity—without changing food type drastically—often leads to weight loss, improved sugars, and better energy within weeks.

> **Example:** A bucket overfilled by a cup every day eventually overflows. The problem is not the bucket—it's repeated excess.

Clinical Example 2: Pancreatic Burnout

In the early stages of overnutrition, the pancreas compensates by producing more insulin. Patients may have normal blood sugar but high insulin levels. Over time, pancreatic beta cells fatigue and fail, leading to overt diabetes. This is not a sudden failure; it is **burnout from chronic overload**.

Ayurveda anticipated this by warning that overeating weakens Agni and produces *Ama* (toxic residue), which blocks metabolic pathways and damages tissues.

> **Example:** Running an engine at maximum RPM may feel powerful, but it shortens engine life dramatically.

4.8.2 Quantity vs Satiety Signals

Modern ultra-processed foods disrupt natural satiety cues. People overeat not because they need more fuel, but because signals of fullness are delayed or ignored. Ayurveda advised eating until **three-quarters full**, leaving space for digestion and movement of gases—an intuitive way to prevent overload.

4.8.3 Clinical correlation:

Eating slowly, stopping before heaviness, and avoiding second servings markedly improve reflux, bloating, and post-meal fatigue.

4.8.4 Special Situations: Illness, Age, and Stress

Digestive capacity drops during illness, after surgery, with aging, and under chronic stress. Yet social habits often encourage "eating to gain strength," which paradoxically worsens weakness by overloading digestion. Light, smaller, frequent meals matched to reduced capacity aid recovery far better than heavy feeding.

Basic Understanding Example:
When a machine is under repair, you reduce load—not increase it.

Preventive Engineering Insight

Fuel quantity is not about restriction; it is about **efficiency**. Matching load to capacity preserves digestion, stabilizes hormones, and prevents toxic accumulation. Overloading—even with "healthy" food—creates waste and disease over time.

4.9 Preventive Fuel Engineering: The Ideal Diet Principle

Preventive fuel engineering focuses on a simple but powerful idea: **the best fuel is not universal—it is appropriate**. In engineering, the ideal fuel is not the most powerful or expensive one, but the one that matches the engine's design, operating conditions, and workload. Similarly, the ideal human diet must match **individual constitution, digestive strength, season, age, mental stress, and lifestyle**. Any diet that ignores these variables may appear healthy on paper but fails in real life.

Ayurveda never promoted rigid food lists or extreme dietary ideologies. Instead, it emphasized **appropriateness and adaptability**. An ideal diet should be fresh, compatible, nourishing, and easy to digest. When these conditions are met, the body naturally maintains weight, energy, immunity, and mental clarity—without constant struggle or medical intervention.

4.9.1 The Four Ayurvedic Principles of Ideal Fuel

Ayurveda summarized the ideal diet in four concise qualities:

- **Hitam (Beneficial):** Food that supports health rather than merely satisfying taste
- **Matram (Adequate):** Quantity appropriate to digestive capacity
- **Snigdham (Unctuous):** Nourishing and lubricating, not dry or depleting
- **Ushnam (Warm):** Supporting digestion and metabolic fire

These principles align closely with modern recommendations favoring whole foods, adequate protein and healthy fats, mindful portions, and warm, freshly cooked meals over cold, processed foods.

4.9.2 Clinical Perspective: Why "Healthy Diets" Sometimes Fail

Clinically, it is common to see patients following "healthy diets" yet suffering from bloating, fatigue, acidity, weight gain, or weakness. The failure often lies not in nutrient content, but in **digestive compatibility**. For example, excessive raw salads may be rich in vitamins but difficult to digest for individuals with weak digestion, leading to gas, nutrient malabsorption, and fatigue. Similarly, very low-fat diets may worsen joint pain, hormonal imbalance, and dryness in some individuals.

Ayurveda would describe this as food being nutritionally rich but **functionally incompatible**.

> **Clinical Example:**
> A middle-aged woman with joint pain and anxiety follows a raw, low-fat diet, believing it to be healthy. Symptoms worsen. Introducing warm, lightly spiced, cooked food with healthy fats improves digestion, joint lubrication, sleep, and mood—without increasing calories.

4.9.3 Seasonal and Environmental Matching

Just as engines require different tuning in winter and summer, the human body requires dietary adjustment with the seasons. Cold seasons demand more warmth and nourishment. Hot seasons require lighter, cooling foods. Ignoring seasonal adaptation leads to allergies, infections, digestive disorders, and metabolic imbalance.

Modern science now recognizes seasonal variation in metabolism, immunity, and gut microbiota—confirming Ayurvedic *Ritucharya* principles.

> **Example:** Using the same engine oil in freezing winters and extreme summers causes damage. Food must also change with the climate.

4.9.4 Digestive Strength Over Nutrition Labels

Preventive fuel engineering prioritizes **digestibility over nutritional theory**. A food that is 100% nutritious but poorly digested becomes a metabolic burden. Ayurveda repeatedly emphasized that digestion (*Agni*) determines whether food becomes nourishment or toxin.

> **Clinical Example:**
> Two patients eat the same balanced meal. One feels energized, the other experiences heaviness and acidity. The difference is digestive strength, not food quality.

> **Example:** Even premium fuel causes problems if the filter is clogged.

4.9.5 Lifestyle Integration: Diet Must Match Daily Load

An ideal diet must also match activity level and stress load. A physically active person requires denser fuel. A sedentary, stressed individual needs lighter, easily digestible meals. Eating heavy food during prolonged sitting or late-night work leads to metabolic congestion.

> **Basic Understanding Example:**
> You don't load a truck the same way when driving uphill and downhill. Load must match effort.

Preventive Engineering Insight

The ideal diet does not fight the body; it **cooperates with it**. When food is beneficial, adequate, nourishing, and warm—matched to person, place, and time—the body self-regulates hunger, weight, energy, and immunity naturally. Disease prevention then becomes effortless rather than forced.

4.10 Key Takeaways: Fuel Determines the Fate of the Machine

The central message of fuel engineering is simple yet profound: **food is not merely nutrition—it is biological instruction**. Every meal delivers information that tells the body how to function, adapt, repair, or deteriorate. Unlike poisons that cause immediate harm, wrong food works silently. It does not destroy the body overnight; it **reprograms physiology gradually**, altering hormones, digestion, immunity, and cellular behavior over years. By the time the disease becomes visible, the programming has already been running for a long time.

Ayurveda reminds us that disease begins much earlier—at the level of digestion, compatibility, timing, quantity, and mental state. This explains why two individuals with similar test results can have very different health trajectories. One may recover quickly with lifestyle correction, while the other progresses to chronic illness. The difference lies in **long-term fueling patterns**, not short-term treatment.

4.10.1 Clinical Perspective: Disease Is Old, Diagnosis Is New

Clinically, patients are often shocked when diagnosed with diabetes, fatty liver, hypertension, or arthritis. They say, "I was fine last year." In reality, the disease process may have started 10–20 years earlier with subtle signs—post-meal sleepiness, mild weight gain, acidity, constipation, fatigue, poor sleep, or stress intolerance. These were early signals of metabolic and digestive strain, ignored because they were not painful or dramatic.

Clinical Example:

A 45-year-old man is diagnosed with type 2 diabetes. He reports years of late dinners, sugary tea multiple times a day, minimal physical activity, and chronic stress. The diabetes did not arrive suddenly; it was **carefully constructed** through daily misfuelling.

4.10.2 Digestion Over Labels: The Forgotten Priority

One of the most important takeaways is that **digestion matters more than nutrition labels**. A food labeled "healthy," "organic," or "high-protein" can still cause disease if it is poorly digested, incompatible, mistimed, or excessive. Ayurveda repeatedly emphasized that even the best food becomes toxic if digestion is weak.

> **Basic Understanding Example:**
> Even premium fuel cannot run an engine with a clogged filter. The problem is not fuel quality alone—it is processing efficiency.

4.10.3 Individual Compatibility: The Missing Link in Modern Diets

Another key lesson is that **individual compatibility is critical**. The same diet can heal one person and harm another. Ignoring individuality leads to predictable disease patterns—obesity in some, inflammation in others, and degeneration in others. This explains why diet trends succeed for a few and fail for many.

> **Clinical Example:**
> Two patients follow the same "high-protein" diet. One improves energy and weight. The other develops acidity, constipation, and kidney strain. The difference is metabolic design, not discipline.

4.10.4 Disease Begins Long Before Symptoms

Symptoms are late-stage events. Long before pain, abnormal scans, or lab reports appear, the body has already been compensating for wrong inputs. During this silent phase, correction is easy and often fully reversible. Once symptoms appear, repair becomes complex, expensive, and sometimes incomplete.

Example: Rust begins inside iron long before it becomes visible. Painting over visible rust does not restore strength.

4.10.5 The Illusion of "Sudden Breakdown"

People often believe a disease is sudden because symptoms appear suddenly. In reality, symptoms are like the final alarm when safety margins are exhausted. The engine did not fail suddenly—it was run on poor fuel, at the wrong timings, in excess quantity, and without maintenance for years.

Example: A bridge collapse looks sudden, but engineers know corrosion and overload existed long before the collapse.

Preventive Engineering Insight

Health is not preserved by occasional detoxes or short-term diets. It is preserved by **daily correct fueling**. Small daily errors accumulate into disease; small daily corrections accumulate into health. Preventive fuel engineering, therefore, focuses not on perfection, but on **consistency**.

Chapter 5

Human Body Servicing Systems: Detoxification, Repair, and Renewal

"If fuel determines performance, waste accumulation determines failure."

5.1 Introduction: Why Servicing is as Important as Fuel

Every engineered system operates under an unavoidable physical law: whenever work is done, waste is generated. A car that runs daily—even on the highest-grade fuel—gradually accumulates carbon deposits inside the engine. Lubricating oil breaks down with heat and friction. Filters clog with dust. Bearings undergo microscopic wear long before they fail visibly. That is why manufacturers insist on periodic servicing. Servicing is not done because the machine has failed; it is done to prevent failure. Ignoring servicing does not stop waste formation—it only allows damage to progress silently until breakdown becomes inevitable.

The human body follows exactly the same engineering principle, but at a vastly higher level of complexity. Every second, billions of biochemical reactions occur inside the body to produce energy, maintain temperature, digest food, transmit nerve signals, repair tissues, and sustain consciousness. These reactions inevitably produce waste substances such as acids, heat, free radicals, metabolic residues, and cellular debris. Digestion leaves undigested remnants, hormonal activity generates breakdown products, and daily exposure to polluted air, contaminated food, chemicals, and psychological stress adds further toxic load. Waste production is therefore **not abnormal—it is a natural consequence of living.**

The real problem begins when **waste removal does not keep pace with waste production.** In machines, this imbalance is prevented by scheduled maintenance. In humans, however, biological servicing is often ignored. People continue eating, working, stressing, and sleeping irregularly while assuming the body will indefinitely "adjust." Early warning signs—such as fatigue, heaviness, poor digestion, skin problems, stiffness, or mental fog—are dismissed as normal or temporary. These are not random discomforts; they are the body's equivalent of a "service required" warning light. When these signals are repeatedly ignored, waste accumulates deeper within tissues and organs.

Unlike machines, the human body does not abruptly shut down at the first sign of overload. It compensates intelligently and silently. Organs work harder, alternative pathways are activated, and symptoms are suppressed. This compensation creates the **illusion of health**, even as internal damage progresses. By the time pain, disease labels, or organ dysfunction appear, the problem is no longer new—the condition is already well established. What appears to be "sudden disease" is actually the final visible stage of years or decades of neglected internal maintenance.

From a preventive medicine perspective, this understanding is critical. **Disease is rarely an accident or a sudden event.** It is the predictable outcome of a long-term imbalance between waste generation and waste elimination. Just as no engineer would expect a machine to perform indefinitely without servicing, it is unreasonable to expect the human body to remain healthy without periodic biological cleaning, repair, and renewal. Recognizing this principle shifts healthcare from crisis management to intelligent maintenance. Servicing the body before breakdown is not optional—it is the most rational and scientific approach to sustaining long-term health.

5.2 Waste Accumulation – The Silent Killer (Expanded)

5.2.1 Sources of Waste in the Human Body

From the viewpoint of modern biomedical science, the human body continuously generates waste as a by-product of living. Every breath taken, every meal digested, and every thought processed at the neurological level produces chemical residues. Normal metabolism generates **reactive oxygen species**, which are highly unstable molecules capable of damaging cells if not neutralized. Excess sugar intake leads to the formation of **advanced glycation end products**, which stiffen tissues and accelerate aging. Chronic mental stress triggers the release of **inflammatory cytokines**, creating a low-grade inflammatory state throughout the body. In addition, daily exposure to pesticides, preservatives, heavy metals, polluted air, and contaminated water adds an external toxic burden that the body must process and eliminate.

Beyond this, digestion itself is a major source of waste when it is inefficient. Poor chewing, irregular eating habits, overeating, incompatible food combinations, and weak digestive power leave behind **undigested food residues**. Altered gut bacteria then act on this residue, producing toxic gases and metabolites that enter circulation. Hormones, once they complete their function, also break down into metabolites that must be neutralized and excreted. When elimination organs such as the liver, intestines, kidneys, skin, and lungs are overloaded or weakened, these wastes begin to accumulate instead of being cleared.

Ayurveda groups all these forms of toxic accumulation under one powerful concept: **Āma**. Āma refers to anything within the body that is **incompletely processed, sticky in nature, obstructive to flow, and harmful to tissues**. Importantly, Āma is not limited to food waste. It includes metabolic toxins, emotional stress residues, and environmental pollutants. Ayurveda emphasizes that even nutritious food can turn into poison if digestion and metabolism are weak.

A simple example clarifies this idea clarifies this idea. If a kitchen is used daily but utensils are never washed properly, layers of sticky grease gradually build up. Even fresh ingredients cooked in those utensils start tasting bad and burn easily. The problem is not the quality of ingredients—it is the failure to clean. Similarly, when digestion and metabolism are impaired, even healthy food contributes to toxin formation instead of nourishment.

5.2.2 How Waste Leads to Disease – An Engineering Analogy

In engineering, every system is designed with a specific **clearance capacity**—the maximum amount of waste or heat it can safely remove while continuing to function. As long as waste generation stays within this limit, the system runs smoothly. The moment waste production exceeds clearance capacity, malfunction begins. The same principle applies to the human body. Disease does not begin when waste appears; it begins when **waste accumulates faster than the body can eliminate it**.

Initially, the body compensates intelligently. Organs work harder, alternative metabolic pathways are activated, and symptoms are suppressed. At this stage, a person may experience vague complaints such as tiredness, heaviness after meals, bloating, mild joint stiffness, dull skin, bad breath, or mental fog. These signs are often ignored because they do not yet interfere with daily life. However, these symptoms are not trivial—they are the body's **early warning signals**, similar to a "service due" light in a vehicle.

When these signals are repeatedly ignored, waste begins to deposit in specific tissues and channels. Blood vessels lose elasticity, lymphatic flow slows, joints accumulate inflammatory debris, gut lining becomes irritated, and cellular communication becomes distorted. In Ayurvedic language, Āma blocks the **Srotas**, or transport channels, disrupting nutrition delivery and waste removal at the tissue level. In modern terms, this translates to chronic inflammation, oxidative stress, insulin resistance, hormonal imbalance, and immune dysregulation.

A simple household analogy makes this process clear. A kitchen sink with a partially blocked drain still allows water to pass, but slowly. Over time, water stagnates, unpleasant odors develop, and bacterial growth increases. Eventually, the sink overflows. The overflow appears sudden, but the blockage developed gradually. In the same way, heart disease, diabetes, arthritis, skin disorders, and autoimmune conditions appear to arise suddenly, but they are the predictable outcome of long-standing waste accumulation and ignored warning signs.

Thus, waste accumulation is called the **silent killer** because it progresses quietly, without dramatic symptoms in the early stages. By the time the disease is diagnosed, the body has already exhausted much of its compensatory capacity. Understanding this principle shifts the focus of health care from treating visible disease to **recognizing and removing waste before irreversible damage occurs**.

5.3 Ayurvedic Servicing Science – Panchakarma

Ayurveda stands apart from all other medical systems because it does not wait for disease to appear before intervening. Instead, it recognizes that **regular internal cleaning is essential for sustaining health**, just as regular servicing is essential for any complex machine. Panchakarma represents this servicing philosophy in a structured, scientific, and repeatable manner. The word Panchakarma refers to **five specialized procedures** designed to remove deeply accumulated waste from the body, re-establish internal balance, and restore the natural intelligence of physiological systems. These procedures are not symbolic or ritualistic; they are practical bio-engineering interventions aimed at clearing the root cause of disease—internal toxic accumulation.

Unlike emergency medical treatments that focus on suppressing symptoms, Panchakarma is a **planned and preventive process**. It is undertaken when the body still has enough strength to tolerate cleansing and respond positively. Ayurveda insists that before deciding any detox procedure, the physician must assess an individual's **Prakriti (body constitution)**, current imbalance, digestive strength, age, seasonal influences, mental state, and disease susceptibility. This ensures that detoxification is not excessive, harmful, or random. In simple terms, Panchakarma is not a "one-size-fits-all" cleanse; it is a **customized servicing schedule**, much like different vehicles require different service protocols based on usage, load, and design.

From a common man's perspective, Panchakarma can be understood as a **deep internal cleaning program** that reaches places where routine daily elimination cannot. Daily bowel movements, urination, sweating, and breathing remove only surface-level waste. Over time, however, toxins settle deeper in tissues such as fat, joints, nerves, and organs. Panchakarma is designed to mobilize this deeply stored waste and safely guide it out through specific elimination routes. This is why people often feel lightness, clarity of mind, improved digestion, and renewed energy after properly conducted Panchakarma—it removes the internal "sludge" that slows down bodily functions.

A simple everyday example makes this clear. Consider a water storage tank at home. Even if clean water flows in daily, sediments slowly settle at the bottom. The water may look clear for months, but eventually, smell, discoloration, or contamination appear. Periodic emptying and scrubbing of the tank is essential to maintain water quality. Panchakarma serves a similar function for the body—it cleanses internal reservoirs before visible contamination manifests as disease.

Another important aspect of Panchakarma is **timing**. Ayurveda recommends detoxification at specific intervals—such as seasonal changes, advancing age, or early stages of imbalance—because these are times when waste accumulation naturally increases. Ignoring these windows leads to deeper disease penetration. Performing Panchakarma early prevents this progression, reduces dependency on long-term medications, and preserves organ function. This preventive approach is what makes Panchakarma a cornerstone of Ayurvedic healthcare rather than a last-resort therapy.

To understand this concept simply, consider automobile servicing. A car may run smoothly and show no immediate problems, yet manufacturers still mandate servicing after a fixed number of kilometers. This is because wear and waste accumulation occur invisibly. Waiting until the engine fails results in costly repairs and permanent damage. Panchakarma follows the same logic. It is performed **before irreversible damage appears**, maintaining the efficiency, longevity, and resilience of the human body. In this way, Panchakarma represents not alternative medicine, but **intelligent preventive engineering applied to human health**.

5.4 Shodhana Vs Shamana – Clean First, Then Repair

Ayurveda approaches treatment with the precision of an engineer who understands that different problems require different strategies. It clearly divides all medical interventions into **Shamana** and **Shodhana**, based on the internal condition of the system. Shamana refers to measures that **pacify symptoms and restore balance without forceful elimination**. This includes medicines, diet regulation, yoga, sleep correction, and lifestyle changes. Shamana works best when the disease is mild, waste accumulation is minimal, and the body's natural clearance systems are still functioning efficiently. In such situations, gentle correction allows the system to self-correct, much like fine-tuning a machine that is still relatively clean.

However, Ayurveda recognizes that many chronic and recurrent diseases do not arise from simple imbalance alone. They arise from **deeply accumulated waste, blockages, and toxic residues** stored within tissues. In these situations, Shamana alone becomes insufficient. This is where **Shodhana**, or deep detoxification, becomes essential. Shodhana actively removes the root cause of disease by eliminating accumulated toxins and clearing blocked pathways. It does not merely calm symptoms; it restores the internal environment in which true healing can occur. Ayurveda, therefore, emphasizes a strict rule: **repair should only follow cleaning**. Attempting to repair a system filled with waste is inefficient and short-lived.

A simple mechanical analogy explains this principle clearly. Imagine an engine that has accumulated thick sludge due to poor maintenance. Adding high-quality engine oil may temporarily reduce noise and friction, giving the impression of improvement. However, the sludge remains inside, continuing to damage internal components. Eventually, the engine overheats or seizes, often more severely than before. In the same way, medicines taken without detoxification may reduce pain, acidity, or inflammation temporarily, but the underlying toxic load remains. Once medication is stopped, symptoms often return—sometimes stronger and more widespread.

From a individual's health perspective, this is commonly seen in everyday illnesses. A person with chronic acidity may take antacids for years, feeling temporary relief each time. However, if the digestive system is clogged with toxins, poor eating habits, and weak metabolism, acidity keeps returning. Another example is joint pain treated repeatedly with painkillers. While pain reduces temporarily, stiffness and degeneration continue silently. Ayurveda interprets this as repeated Shamana without prior Shodhana. The symptoms are controlled, but the disease mechanism remains active.

Shodhana is therefore not an aggressive or extreme approach—it is a **logical preparatory step**. By removing accumulated waste first, Shodhana restores the body's responsiveness. After detoxification, even small doses of medicines, proper diet, and lifestyle changes become highly effective. This is why Ayurveda often prescribes Shodhana once or periodically, followed by Shamana for maintenance. The sequence is crucial. Cleaning the internal environment first ensures that nourishment, medicines, and regenerative therapies can reach tissues effectively and produce lasting results.

In simple terms, Shamana is like routine maintenance—adjusting settings, adding lubrication, and correcting usage habits—while Shodhana is like a complete internal cleaning and overhaul. Both are essential, but their order matters. Ayurveda's timeless warning, "Do not repair without cleaning," reflects deep biological wisdom. Ignoring this principle leads to recurrent disease, drug dependence, and gradual loss of vitality. Following it leads to sustainable healing, resilience, and long-term health preservation.

5.5 The Five Servicing Systems (Pancha Karma)

5.5.1 The Five Servicing Systems (pancha Karma) – Expanded Explanation

Ayurveda views the human body as a complex, self-regulating machine that requires **different servicing tools for different systems**. Just as an engineer uses separate mechanisms to clean fuel lines, cooling systems, wiring circuits, and hydraulic units, Ayurveda designed **five distinct detoxification procedures**, collectively known as Panchakarma. Each procedure targets a specific zone of waste accumulation, a dominant physiological imbalance (Dosha), and a particular route of elimination. These are not interchangeable therapies; each has a precise role in restoring functional balance.

Vamana (therapeutic emesis) is designed to remove excess heaviness, mucus, and stagnation associated with Kapha dominance. When Kapha accumulates, it slows metabolism, clogs airways, and promotes fat deposition and insulin resistance. Vamana cleanses the upper digestive tract and respiratory channels, relieving congestion and restoring metabolic clarity. From a common mom's point of view, it functions like draining excess water from a flooded engine compartment—until the excess is removed, the engine cannot breathe or perform efficiently. Clinically, patients with obesity, asthma, allergies, or early metabolic disorders often feel immediate lightness, improved breathing, and better appetite control after proper Vamana, provided it is followed by a disciplined diet and lifestyle correction.

Virechana (therapeutic purgation) focuses on cleansing the liver–gut axis, where heat, acidity, and toxins related to Pitta accumulate. The liver acts as the body's primary chemical processing plant, and when overloaded, toxins spill into circulation, affecting skin, blood, and digestion. Virechana removes this excess heat and restores smooth bile flow and gut–liver communication. In simple engineering terms, it is like cleaning a blocked oil circulation system—once oil flows freely, overheating and friction reduce automatically. Patients suffering from acidity, skin disorders, fatty liver, or inflammatory conditions often experience a sense of internal cooling, improved digestion, clearer skin, and mental calm after Virechana.

Basti (medicated enema) is considered the most powerful of all Panchakarma procedures because it directly addresses Vata, the principle governing movement, nerve function, circulation, and degeneration. The colon is the main seat of Vata, and disturbances here affect joints, muscles, nerves, and even mental stability. Modern understanding recognizes the colon as a hub of the gut microbiome and the enteric nervous system. Basti therapies modulate inflammation, calm nerve signaling, and improve tissue nourishment. From a common man's perspective, Basti works like repairing the central wiring of a machine—if wiring is faulty, no component works properly. This is why patients with arthritis, back pain, neurological complaints, or degenerative disorders often experience long-lasting relief and improved mobility after structured Basti cycles.

Nasya (nasal therapy) addresses disorders of the head and neck region, including the brain, sinuses, sense organs, and hormonal regulation centers. Ayurveda recognizes the nose as the gateway to the head, and modern science confirms direct nose-to-brain pathways influencing circulation and neuroendocrine function. Nasya removes accumulated toxins, excess mucus, and stagnation from cranial channels. In simple mechanical terms, it is like cleaning the control panel and sensors of a machine—accurate signals ensure smooth and coordinated functioning. Patients with migraine, sinusitis, anxiety, cervical stiffness, or sleep disturbances often report mental clarity, improved breathing, and reduced head-related symptoms after Nasya.

Raktamokshana (blood detoxification) is a localized cleansing procedure used when toxins are concentrated in the blood and microcirculation. Chronic inflammation, skin diseases, varicose veins, and localized swelling often indicate stagnant or contaminated blood flow. Raktamokshana removes this toxic load, allowing fresh circulation and tissue healing. From a layman's perspective, it is similar to releasing contaminated coolant from a specific part of a system—if not removed, corrosion and overheating continue despite other repairs. Patients frequently notice a rapid reduction in redness, pain, itching, and swelling after appropriate blood detoxification.

Together, these five servicing systems form a **complete internal maintenance protocol**. They do not merely suppress disease; they restore flow, clarity, and intelligence to the body's systems. When applied judiciously, at the right time and in the right individual, Panchakarma prevents disease progression, enhances recovery, and preserves long-term functional health.

5.6 Poorva Karma – Preparing The Machine

In any field of engineering, preparation is considered as important as the actual repair. No skilled engineer attempts to service a machine that is cold, dry, and rigid, because such an approach risks incomplete cleaning and structural damage. Machines are first warmed, lubricated, and gradually brought into an optimal state so that internal deposits can be loosened and removed safely. Ayurveda applies this same intelligent principle to the human body through **Poorva Karma**, the preparatory phase before detoxification. Poorva Karma ensures that the body is receptive, flexible, and physiologically ready for effective waste removal.

Ayurveda achieves this preparation through two fundamental procedures: **Snehan (oleation)** and **Swedana (sudation)**. Snehan involves internal and external lubrication using oils or fats suited to the individual's constitution and condition. At a biological level, Snehan softens tissues, improves cellular flexibility, and mobilizes toxins that are tightly bound within fat, joints, and connective tissues. Many toxins are fat-soluble and remain trapped deep inside the body unless adequate lubrication is provided. In simple terms, Snehan works like applying oil to rusted bolts—without lubrication, the bolts resist movement and may break; with oil, they loosen smoothly and safely.

Swedana follows Snehan and uses controlled heat to induce sweating. Heat dilates channels, increases circulation, and accelerates metabolic activity, allowing loosened toxins to move from deeper tissues toward the digestive tract for elimination. From engineering perspective, Swedana functions like warming hardened grease before cleaning it. Cold grease is stiff and resistant, but when warmed, it melts and flows easily. Similarly, toxins that are immobile and stuck within tissues begin to flow once heat and circulation increase, making detoxification efficient and less stressful for the body.

Poorva Karma also plays a crucial protective role. Sudden detoxification without preparation can shock the system, leading to weakness, dizziness, or incomplete elimination. By gradually loosening toxins and opening pathways, Snehan and Swedana reduce strain on elimination organs such as the liver, intestines, and kidneys. This staged approach reflects deep physiological wisdom—**the body is not forced to cleanse; it is guided to release waste naturally**. As a result, detoxification becomes smoother, safer, and more complete.

A simple everyday example makes this concept clear. Imagine trying to clean burned food from a dry pan using force alone—it requires excessive effort and may damage the surface. If the pan is first soaked in warm water and oil, the residue loosens and can be removed effortlessly. Poorva Karma performs this "soaking" function for the body. By the time the main Panchakarma procedures are administered, toxins are already mobilized, channels are open, and elimination pathways are active.

Thus, Poorva Karma is not an optional ritual but a **scientific preparation phase** that determines the success of detoxification. It reflects the Ayurvedic understanding that effective cleansing depends not only on what is removed, but **how and when it is removed**. Proper preparation ensures that detoxification is thorough, safe, and restorative rather than exhausting. In the engineering language of the body, Poorva Karma is the essential step that transforms detoxification from a risky intervention into a precise and intelligent servicing process.

5.7 Modern Detox Myths Vs Ayurvedic Reality

In recent years, the idea of "detox" has become popular in mainstream culture, often promoted through juice cleanses, herbal teas, powders, fasting challenges, or dietary supplements. These methods promise rapid cleansing, weight loss, glowing skin, and renewed energy within a few days. While attractive in theory, most modern detox trends are based on **simplistic assumptions** about the human body. They assume that toxins are superficial, uniform in everyone, and easily removable through short-term dietary changes. In reality, the human body is a complex biological system where toxins accumulate at different depths, in different tissues, and through different mechanisms. A one-method-for-all approach ignores this complexity.

One major myth of modern detox programs is the belief that **quick cleansing equals deep cleansing**. Drinking juices or consuming supplements may temporarily reduce calorie intake or give the digestive system a short rest, leading to a brief feeling of lightness. However, this effect is often mistaken for detoxification. In many cases, such methods only reduce digestive workload temporarily without removing deeply stored waste from tissues such as fat, joints, nerves, or organs. Once normal eating resumes, symptoms often return. This is similar to skipping meals to feel lighter—relief is temporary, not corrective.

Another critical limitation of modern detox trends is the **lack of personalization**. People of different ages, body types, digestive capacities, stress levels, and disease tendencies are advised to follow the same detox plan. In engineering terms, this is like applying the same servicing protocol to a motorcycle, a truck, and an aircraft engine. What benefits one system may damage another. Some individuals become weak, dizzy, anxious, or develop digestive disturbances after aggressive detox programs because their bodies were not prepared or suited for such interventions. Ayurveda recognizes that detoxification without considering individual constitution can create more imbalance than benefit.

Modern detox methods also frequently ignore **the importance of supervision and sequencing**. Many people attempt detox while continuing stressful work schedules, poor sleep, and mental overload. This places additional strain on the nervous and hormonal systems. Ayurveda, in contrast, insists that detoxification must be supervised, gradual, and properly timed. Preparation (Poorva Karma), main cleansing (Pradhana Karma), and recovery (Paschat Karma) are all considered essential. Skipping preparation or recovery is like dismantling an engine without warming it up or reassembling it without testing—damage becomes likely.

Panchakarma succeeds because it is **systematic and biologically logical**. It recognizes that toxins are not floating freely in the bloodstream waiting to be flushed out. They are often lodged in tissues, bound to fat, stuck in channels, or circulating repeatedly due to impaired metabolism. Panchakarma first loosens these toxins, then guides them toward specific elimination routes, and finally restores strength and balance after removal. This stepwise approach respects the body's physiology rather than forcing abrupt changes.

A simple everyday example highlights this contrast clearly. Washing the exterior of a car may make it look clean and shiny, but it does nothing to remove carbon deposits inside the engine, sludge in oil lines, or debris in filters. Over time, the car will still break down despite its clean appearance. Panchakarma is equivalent to opening the hood and cleaning the engine, fuel system, and internal components. It addresses the **root of the problem**, not just the surface.

Another useful analogy is house cleaning. Spraying air freshener may temporarily mask unpleasant odors, but it does not remove garbage hidden under furniture or in corners. True cleaning requires identifying the source of dirt, removing it, and then restoring order. Modern detox trends often act like air fresheners—temporary and cosmetic. Panchakarma functions like deep cleaning, restoring hygiene at the source.

In essence, the Ayurvedic reality of detoxification is grounded in **depth, discrimination, and discipline**. It does not promise instant results, but it delivers lasting change. It treats detoxification not as a fashionable shortcut, but as a serious medical process that requires planning, expertise, and respect for individual biology. By understanding this difference, one can see why Panchakarma has survived for thousands of years as a preventive and therapeutic system, while most modern detox fads disappear as quickly as they arise.

5.8 Post-Servicing – Renewal & Rejuvenation

Once detoxification is completed, the human body enters a unique physiological state that Ayurveda describes as **heightened receptivity**. During this phase, channels are clear, metabolic waste has been removed, digestion is stronger, and cellular communication is restored. Just as a thoroughly cleaned machine responds better to lubrication and fine-tuning, the cleansed body responds more effectively to nourishment and rebuilding therapies. Ayurveda emphasizes that detoxification alone is not the final goal; it is the **foundation upon which true repair and renewal become possible**.

Rasayana therapy represents this phase of rebuilding and rejuvenation. Rasayana does not merely add strength superficially; it improves the quality of tissues at a fundamental level. After detox, nutrients, medicines, and lifestyle interventions reach deeper tissues more efficiently because internal blockages have been removed. Immunity improves, energy levels stabilize, mental clarity increases, and recovery from illness becomes faster. In Simple terms, it is like replacing worn-out machine parts after cleaning the engine—performance does not just return to baseline, it often exceeds previous levels.

A key concept in this phase is **tissue intelligence restoration**. When waste accumulates, tissues become confused in their function—repair slows, immunity weakens, and aging accelerates. After detoxification, Rasayana therapies help tissues "remember" how to function correctly. For example, muscles regain strength, joints regain lubrication, nerves regain stability, and the digestive system regains rhythm. This is why people often feel younger, lighter, and more resilient after proper post-detox care, even without dramatic external changes.

A simple everyday example explains this clearly. Consider an old appliance that has been clogged with dust and debris. Cleaning alone improves function, but replacing worn belts, lubricating moving parts, and recalibrating controls dramatically extend its lifespan. Similarly, Rasayana therapies nourish tissues that have been depleted by stress, poor diet, illness, or aging. This nourishment is not excessive; it is precise and targeted, ensuring that repair happens without creating new imbalances.

Another important aspect of post-servicing care is **stabilization**. After deep cleansing, the body is sensitive and adaptable. If proper recovery measures are ignored, old habits can quickly recreate imbalance. Rasayana therapy, along with disciplined diet, rest, and lifestyle regulation, helps stabilize gains achieved through detoxification. In engineering terms, this is similar to testing and running-in an overhauled engine under controlled conditions before returning it to full load. This phase prevents relapse and ensures long-term benefits.

Post-servicing rejuvenation also plays a critical role in **slowing biological aging**. Accumulated toxins accelerate wear at the cellular level, leading to premature aging and chronic disease. By removing these toxins and then rebuilding tissues with Rasayana therapy, the rate of degeneration slows. People often notice improved skin texture, better sleep, enhanced memory, stronger immunity, and reduced susceptibility to illness. These changes are not cosmetic; they reflect deeper physiological renewal.

In essence, post-servicing is where healing becomes sustainable. Detoxification clears the path, but rejuvenation determines how far the body can travel afterward. Without renewal, detox remains incomplete; without detox, renewal is ineffective. Ayurveda integrates both into a single intelligent system. Just as a machine's longevity depends not only on cleaning but also on timely replacement and reinforcement of parts, human longevity and vitality depend on **systematic detoxification followed by thoughtful rejuvenation**. This balanced approach transforms healthcare from short-term symptom control into long-term preservation of health, function, and quality of life.

5.9 Preventive Servicing – The Missing Link

Preventive servicing is one of the most powerful yet most neglected principles in modern healthcare. Ayurveda clearly states that **health must be maintained before disease appears**, not merely repaired after damage occurs. Just as machines are serviced at fixed intervals regardless of whether they show visible faults, Ayurveda recommends **seasonal, age-specific, and condition-specific detoxification even in apparently healthy individuals**. The goal is not to treat illness, but to prevent the internal conditions that eventually give rise to illness. This approach recognizes that imbalance and waste accumulation begin long before symptoms are felt.

Seasonal changes are a major reason why preventive servicing is necessary. Each season places a unique stress on the body. Heat accumulates in summer, dryness increases in winter, and congestion builds during rainy seasons. Ayurveda observed that these seasonal influences naturally promote waste accumulation and Dosha imbalance. Preventive detox at seasonal junctions clears this buildup before it settles deep into tissues. In simple terms, this is like servicing a vehicle before extreme weather conditions—checking coolant before summer or lubricating parts before winter prevents breakdown under stress.

Age-specific preventive servicing is equally important. As the body ages, digestion weakens, metabolism slows, and waste clearance becomes less efficient. Childhood, adulthood, and old age each have distinct physiological vulnerabilities. Ayurveda recommends gentle and appropriate detoxification at different life stages to maintain functional balance. A layman's analogy is the difference between maintaining a new machine versus an old one. An older system needs more frequent inspection and careful servicing to keep it running smoothly. Ignoring this leads to rapid deterioration and frequent repairs.

Preventive servicing also applies to individuals with **disease tendencies**, even if they are currently symptom-free. A person with a family history of diabetes, heart disease, arthritis, or skin disorders may appear healthy for years, yet internally carry a higher risk of waste accumulation in specific systems. Ayurveda addresses this proactively through targeted detox and lifestyle correction. This is similar to reinforcing a bridge known to carry heavy traffic—strengthening it early prevents collapse later.

From a practical standpoint, preventive servicing dramatically reduces long-term healthcare costs and medication dependency. Chronic diseases often require lifelong drug use once established. Preventive detoxification reduces disease incidence, delays onset, and lowers severity, thereby decreasing the need for prolonged medication. In everyday terms, **routine servicing costs far less than emergency repairs**. Fixing a small issue early prevents catastrophic failure later, saving time, money, and suffering.

A simple daily-life example illustrates this clearly. Regular dental cleaning prevents cavities and gum disease. Waiting until pain appears often means root canal treatment or tooth extraction. The same logic applies to the entire body. Preventive servicing keeps systems clean, responsive, and resilient. Emergency treatment, on the other hand, is reactive, expensive, and often incomplete.

Preventive servicing also preserves **quality of life**, not just longevity. Individuals who undergo periodic detox and maintenance often experience better energy, clearer thinking, stronger immunity, improved digestion, and emotional stability. They fall sick less often, recover faster, and age more gracefully. These benefits arise not from aggressive intervention, but from **respecting the body's maintenance requirements**.

In essence, preventive servicing is the missing link between health and disease. Modern medicine excels at emergency repair, while Ayurveda excels at intelligent maintenance. When preventive servicing is ignored, healthcare becomes crisis-driven. When it is embraced, health becomes sustainable. Just as regular servicing prevents accidents and prolongs machine life, **preventive biological servicing preserves human vitality, reduces disease burden, and transforms healthcare from reactive to proactive**.

5.10 Key Take-Home Principles

The first and most important principle is that **disease is not bad luck or sudden misfortune**. From an engineering and biological perspective, disease is the logical outcome of **gradual waste accumulation combined with delayed servicing**. The body gives repeated warning signals—fatigue, poor digestion, stiffness, disturbed sleep, irritability, or frequent infections—but these are often ignored or normalized. Just as a machine fails after prolonged neglect rather than random chance, the human body breaks down when internal waste exceeds its capacity to compensate. Understanding this removes fear and helplessness from disease and replaces them with responsibility and predictability.

The second principle is that **detoxification is a biological necessity**, not an alternative belief or cultural ritual. Every living system must eliminate waste to survive. The liver, kidneys, intestines, lungs, and skin are natural detox organs, but when their load exceeds capacity, additional support becomes essential. Ayurveda simply formalized this necessity into a structured medical system. A simple example is is household garbage disposal. Removing waste daily is not optional or belief-based—it is essential for hygiene. Ignoring it leads inevitably to disease, irrespective of beliefs.

The third principle clarifies that **Panchakarma is scientific biological engineering**, not ritualistic practice. Its methods are based on observation of physiology, elimination pathways, tissue behavior, and seasonal influence. Each procedure has a specific target, timing, and mechanism. When performed correctly, Panchakarma follows the same logic as engineering overhauls—identify accumulation, loosen it, remove it safely, and restore function. Calling it a ritual is similar to calling engine servicing superstition, simply because it was practiced before modern machines existed.

The fourth principle emphasizes that **repair without detox leads to recurrence**. Treating symptoms without removing the underlying waste is like repainting a rusted structure without removing corrosion.

The surface may look improved, but damage continues underneath. This explains why many chronic diseases return repeatedly despite medication. Painkillers may suppress pain, antacids may suppress acidity, and steroids may suppress inflammation, but unless the internal toxic load is reduced, disease mechanisms remain active. Detox creates the internal environment necessary for lasting repair.

The fifth principle redefines prevention. **Prevention is not fear-driven medicine**—it is intelligent maintenance. Preventive servicing is done not because one is afraid of disease, but because one understands how systems function over time. Regular oil changes are not performed out of fear of accidents; they are done to ensure smooth performance and longevity. Similarly, preventive detox and lifestyle correction are acts of wisdom, not anxiety. They reflect respect for the body's design limits.

Another key understanding is that **early intervention is always gentler than late intervention**. Removing small amounts of waste periodically requires minimal effort and causes little discomfort. Waiting until waste accumulates deeply requires aggressive treatment and carries a higher risk. This is why Ayurveda emphasizes seasonal and age-appropriate servicing rather than emergency detox during severe disease. In everyday terms, cleaning a lightly dusty room is easy; cleaning a house neglected for years is exhausting.

These principles also highlight the difference between **health maintenance and disease management**. Disease management focuses on controlling symptoms after damage has occurred. Health maintenance focuses on preserving optimal function before damage begins. Panchakarma, when used preventively, belongs to the second category. It keeps systems clean, responsive, and resilient, reducing the need for long-term medication and invasive procedures.

Finally, these take-home principles shift healthcare from a reactive model to a **predictive and preventive model**. Instead of asking "Why did this disease happen to me?", the better question becomes "What accumulated inside me, and for how long?" This shift empowers individuals and physicians alike. It transforms medicine from crisis response to intelligent stewardship of the human body.

In summary, the essence of these principles is simple yet profound: **the body is an intelligent machine that thrives on regular maintenance**. Waste accumulation is inevitable, but disease is not. When servicing is timely, detoxification is scientific, repair follows cleaning, and prevention becomes routine, health is no longer fragile—it becomes sustainable.

Chapter 6

Stress Engineering: Load Management in the Human Machine

6.1 Introduction: When Load Exceeds Design Capacity

In engineering science, stress is defined as the load applied to a structure in relation to its inherent strength and design tolerance. Every bridge, engine, dam, or building is created with a clear understanding of how much weight, pressure, vibration, and environmental force it can safely handle. When these limits are respected, the structure performs efficiently for decades. However, when load repeatedly exceeds design capacity—whether due to overuse, neglect, or poor planning—the damage does not appear instantly. Microscopic cracks begin to form, materials lose elasticity, joints loosen, and efficiency slowly declines. What appears to be a sudden collapse is almost always the final stage of a long, silent process of accumulated overload. Engineers know that failure is rarely an accident; it is the delayed recognition of excessive stress.

The human body obeys the same universal law of load and capacity. Although it is the most advanced biological machine ever known, capable of self-repair and adaptation, it is not designed for infinite strain. The difference between machines and humans lies in how stress is applied and detected. Machines have gauges, alarms, and automatic shutdown systems. The human body, however, is exposed to continuous and often invisible stressors—mental pressure from work, emotional strain from relationships, irregular eating habits, sleep deprivation, chronic inflammation, social insecurity, and nonstop sensory stimulation. There is no loud alarm that forces a shutdown. People continue to work, socialize, and perform daily responsibilities, appearing functional and productive, while internal systems quietly bear increasing load beyond safe limits.

This hidden overload explains why many individuals feel "fine" for years before suddenly being diagnosed with a chronic disease. Just as a bridge may look intact while its internal steel framework is corroding, the human body may appear normal while internal regulatory systems are weakening. The nervous system remains constantly activated, hormones are repeatedly pushed out of balance, digestion becomes inefficient, and immunity loses precision. Because the damage accumulates gradually, the body adapts by compensating. These compensations create the illusion of health, even as reserve capacity steadily diminishes.

Modern diseases must therefore be understood as outcomes of long-term overload rather than random events. Conditions such as hypertension, diabetes, heart disease, autoimmune disorders, chronic digestive problems, and depression are biological equivalents of metal fatigue and system breakdown. They do not arise overnight. Just as metal repeatedly bent eventually snaps, tissues repeatedly stressed eventually lose resilience. Modern medicine often focuses on the final failure point, while ignoring the years of excessive load that preceded it.

Ayurveda recognized this principle centuries ago, long before the language of engineering existed. It identified excessive physical effort, emotional strain, fear, grief, anger, worry, and suppression of natural bodily urges as direct causes of disease. These factors were understood as forces that disturb internal balance and overload physiological systems. By continuously pushing the body beyond its adaptive capacity, they weaken digestion, disturb circulation, deplete tissues, and impair mental stability. In modern terms, Ayurveda was describing chronic stress load and its systemic consequences.

Stress, therefore, is not merely an emotional feeling or a psychological inconvenience. It is a real, measurable mechanical load acting on the body's control systems. It alters nervous signaling, disrupts hormonal rhythms, weakens immune coordination, and distorts metabolism. A simple example illustrates this clearly. Consider a water pump designed to operate for eight hours a day. If it is forced to run continuously without rest, it may still pump water for some time, but internal parts will overheat, lubrication will fail, and wear will accelerate. One day, the pump suddenly stops working. The failure seems sudden, but the cause was continuous overuse without recovery.

Similarly, the human body can tolerate occasional stress and even grow stronger from it. However, when stress becomes constant and recovery is absent, capacity declines. Sleep becomes poor, digestion weakens, energy drops, and minor complaints slowly turn into major illnesses. Disease is not the beginning of the problem; it is the final visible signal that design limits were crossed repeatedly and for too long. Understanding health through this lens shifts the focus from emergency repair to intelligent load management, timely rest, and preventive maintenance of the human machine.

6.2 Engineering Definition of Stress vs Biological Stress

In engineering, stress has a precise and measurable meaning. When a load is applied to any structure—such as weight on a bridge, pressure inside a pipe, or torque on an engine shaft—the material experiences internal strain. If this load is occasional and within design limits, the structure returns to its original state. However, when the same load is applied repeatedly, or when the load exceeds capacity, deformation begins. At first, this deformation may be microscopic and invisible, but over time, it progresses into fatigue, wear, and loss of strength. Bearings slowly grind down, engine efficiency drops, and structural joints loosen. Engineers know that most mechanical failures are not sudden events; they are the final stage of long-term stress that was tolerated for too long.

The human body follows an identical principle, but the process occurs through biological pathways rather than metal and mechanics.

When a person experiences stress—whether mental, emotional, physical, or metabolic—the nervous system is the first to respond. Stress signals activate the brain, which then influences hormone release, blood sugar regulation, immune activity, digestion, and circulation. Initially, the body adapts efficiently. It raises energy levels, sharpens attention, and temporarily sacrifices non-essential functions to cope with demand. This adaptive phase is similar to a machine temporarily running at higher RPM to meet a short-term workload.

Problems arise when stress becomes continuous and recovery is absent. Just as a machine cannot run permanently in overload mode, the human body cannot remain in a heightened stress state indefinitely. Over time, stress hormones remain elevated, digestion becomes inefficient, immunity loses precision, and metabolism shifts toward inflammation and energy conservation. These changes gradually distort normal physiology. The result is not one isolated malfunction but a pattern of chronic disease. High blood pressure, diabetes, autoimmune disorders, irritable bowel syndrome, depression, and heart disease emerge as different expressions of the same underlying problem: prolonged systemic overload.

A simple example clarifies this process. Imagine a ceiling fan designed to run for a few hours at a time. If it is forced to run continuously at maximum speed, the motor heats up, lubrication dries, noise increases, and eventually the fan stops working. The failure does not occur on the first day; it happens after months or years of excessive use. Similarly, a human being may handle intense work, emotional strain, or poor lifestyle habits for some time. The body compensates by drawing on reserves. But continuous stress gradually exhausts these reserves, leading to visible illness.

The most important difference between machines and humans lies in the pattern of failure. Machines usually fail locally. A car may have a faulty gearbox while the engine, brakes, and electrical system remain intact. Repairing or replacing the damaged part restores function. In contrast, the human body fails systemically. Because stress acts on the nervous and hormonal control centers, it disrupts multiple organs at once. A stressed individual often develops sleep problems, digestive disturbances, hormonal imbalance, emotional instability, weakened immunity, and chronic pain simultaneously. Treating one organ alone does not solve the problem, because the root cause lies in system-wide overload.

Another everyday example can be seen in electrical systems. If one appliance is overloaded, it may burn out without affecting others. But if the main power supply fluctuates or is overloaded, multiple appliances fail together. Stress in the human body behaves like a disturbance in the main power supply. It affects brain signaling, hormone coordination, immune response, and cellular energy production all at once. Therefore, biological stress cannot be understood or treated as an isolated problem. It must be recognized as a systemic engineering failure caused by prolonged load beyond design capacity.

Understanding stress through this engineering lens changes how disease is viewed. Illness is no longer seen as a sudden enemy or a random defect. It becomes the predictable outcome of long-standing overload without adequate rest, repair, or maintenance. Just as engineers prevent machine failure by monitoring load and allowing recovery, human health depends on recognizing stress early and restoring balance before systemic breakdown occurs.

6.3 The Stress Response: The Body's Emergency Engineering System

From a modern scientific standpoint, stress activates a powerful survival mechanism known as the hypothalamic-pituitary-adrenal (HPA) axis, which functions as the body's emergency control system. When the brain perceives any form of threat—physical danger, emotional pressure, time urgency, or even constant worry—it sends signals to the adrenal glands to release stress hormones such as cortisol, adrenaline, and noradrenaline. These hormones rapidly prepare the body for action by increasing heart rate, raising blood pressure, mobilizing glucose for instant energy, sharpening attention, and temporarily suppressing non-essential functions like digestion and reproduction. This response is not harmful by nature; in fact, it is essential for survival and has protected humans for thousands of years.

Short-term stress is therefore adaptive and beneficial. It allows a person to react quickly in emergencies, meet deadlines, escape danger, or perform under pressure. A simple layman's example is pressing the accelerator briefly while overtaking another vehicle. The engine revs higher, fuel consumption increases, and the system works harder—but only for a short time. Once the task is completed, the accelerator is released, and the engine returns to normal cruising speed. In the same way, after short-term stress, the body is designed to return to a calm, balanced state where repair, digestion, and recovery can occur.

The problem arises when this emergency mode remains switched on continuously. Modern life rarely provides true shutdown or recovery. Work deadlines, financial worries, job insecurity, relationship conflicts, constant notifications, late-night screen exposure, poor sleep, and irregular meals repeatedly activate the stress response. The body is unable to distinguish between a real physical threat and a mental or emotional one, so it responds to both in the same way. As a result, many individuals live in a constant state of low-grade alarm, with stress hormones circulating throughout the day and night.

An engineering analogy explains this situation clearly. Emergency diesel generators are designed to operate only during power failures. They provide temporary support until normal power is restored. If a factory begins running daily on emergency generators, fuel consumption rises sharply, engines overheat, noise increases, lubrication fails, and maintenance costs escalate. Eventually, the generator breaks down completely. Similarly, the human stress response is meant for emergencies, not for daily life. When cortisol and adrenaline are released continuously, the body's systems begin to suffer from overuse and exhaustion.

Chronic activation of stress hormones produces predictable biological consequences. Persistently high cortisol raises blood sugar levels, leading to insulin resistance and eventually diabetes. Adrenaline keeps blood pressure elevated, contributing to hypertension and heart disease. The immune system becomes confused—sometimes suppressed, leading to frequent infections, and sometimes overactive, leading to autoimmune disorders. Digestion weakens, causing acidity, bloating, constipation, or irritable bowel syndrome. Brain functions such as memory, focus, and emotional stability decline, resulting in anxiety, depression, and burnout. These are not separate diseases; they are different expressions of the same chronic emergency state.

A common example can be seen in daily work life. A person under constant pressure may rely on caffeine to stay alert, skip meals due to deadlines, and sacrifice sleep to complete tasks. Initially, productivity seems high. Over months or years, however, fatigue sets in, concentration drops, mood becomes unstable, and illnesses appear. The body, like an overheated engine, begins to lose efficiency despite running harder. What appears as laziness or weakness is actually system exhaustion.

Another simple comparison is with mobile phone usage. A phone performs well during occasional heavy use, such as during an important call or navigation. But if multiple apps run continuously, brightness remains high, and the phone is never allowed to rest or cool, battery life shortens, heating increases, and performance slows. Likewise, the human body can handle short periods of intense stress but deteriorates when stress becomes a permanent operating condition.

Thus, the stress response is not the enemy; misuse of the stress response is the real problem. The emergency engineering system of the body saves life in the short term, but damages health when used without rest. Modern humans are not truly living in a balanced state; they are continuously coping, compensating, and surviving. Without deliberate recovery, relaxation, and restoration, this chronic emergency mode inevitably leads to physical, mental, and emotional breakdown.

6.4 Ayurveda's Stress Engineering Model

Ayurveda approaches stress as a disturbance in the body's fundamental regulatory force known as Vata. Vata is responsible for all movement and communication within the body, including nerve impulses, breathing, circulation of blood, transportation of nutrients, elimination of waste, and mental activity such as thinking and decision-making. In simple terms, Vata functions like the control wiring and signal transmission system of a complex machine. When this system operates smoothly, coordination between different parts of the body is effortless. When it becomes disturbed, confusion and malfunction spread throughout the entire system. Stress, according to Ayurveda, is one of the most powerful forces that destabilizes this control network.

Chronic stress particularly affects specific functional aspects of Vata. Prana Vata governs breathing, sensory perception, attention, and mental calmness. Under constant stress, breathing becomes shallow, the mind becomes restless, and sleep quality deteriorates. Udana Vata controls effort, speech, confidence, enthusiasm, and motivation. When stressed, individuals often feel mentally drained, lose initiative, struggle to express themselves clearly, and feel exhausted even after resting. Vyana Vata governs circulation and coordinated movement throughout the body. Disturbance here leads to poor circulation, palpitations, muscle tightness, tremors, and generalized body aches. These changes explain why stress affects not just emotions but breathing patterns, speech, posture, and physical stamina.

When stress continues without relief, Vata becomes excessive and erratic, similar to an electrical system exposed to fluctuating voltage. This instability directly impairs Agni, the digestive and metabolic fire responsible for converting food into usable energy. Digestion becomes irregular—sometimes weak, sometimes overly sensitive, but rarely balanced. Food may be eaten in sufficient quantity, yet it is not properly digested or absorbed. As a result, partially processed material accumulates in the body as Ama, which can be understood as metabolic waste or internal toxins. A simple example is a stove with an unsteady flame; even good-quality food cannot cook properly, leading to undercooked, indigestible meals.

Over time, the presence of Ama and disturbed digestion leads to gradual depletion of body tissues, a process Ayurveda calls Dhatu kshaya. Muscles lose strength, joints lose lubrication, skin becomes dry, hair thins, immunity weakens, and mental endurance declines. The person may feel constantly tired but unable to rest, mentally overactive yet physically exhausted. Common complaints such as dryness, constipation, bloating, joint stiffness, anxiety, fearfulness, and forgetfulness are early signs of this process. These symptoms are not isolated problems; they are warning signals that the body's stress load has exceeded its adaptive capacity.

Ayurveda clearly identifies emotional factors such as worry, grief, fear, and anger as direct aggravators of Vata. This explains why emotional stress often first appears as physical symptoms rather than as obvious disease. For example, a person undergoing prolonged emotional strain may develop insomnia, poor appetite, irregular bowel habits, neck or back pain, and menstrual irregularities. These symptoms arise even when medical tests appear normal. Just as a machine with disturbed control circuitry shows erratic performance before breaking down, the body shows functional disturbances long before structural disease appears.

If stress continues unchecked, deeper systems become involved. Hormonal rhythms lose stability, immunity becomes confused, and tissue repair slows down. Degenerative conditions such as osteoarthritis, neurological disorders, premature aging, and autoimmune diseases become more likely. Ayurveda explains this progression by showing how prolonged Vata disturbance spreads from functional imbalance to structural damage. What begins as restlessness and poor sleep eventually manifests as chronic disease, much like repeated vibration in a machine eventually leads to cracked components.

A simple everyday example helps clarify this model. During travel or major life changes, people often experience dryness, constipation, fatigue, anxiety, and disturbed sleep. These are temporary expressions of Vata aggravation caused by irregular routine and mental strain. Once routine, rest, and nourishment are restored, balance returns. However, when such irregularity becomes a permanent lifestyle—irregular meals, constant worry, poor sleep, and mental overload—the temporary imbalance turns into chronic pathology. Ayurveda's stress engineering model emphasizes that disease is not sudden; it is the predictable result of prolonged disturbance in the body's primary regulatory system.

In this way, Ayurveda presents stress as a tangible physiological force rather than a vague emotional concept. Stress directly disrupts movement, digestion, circulation, tissue nourishment, and mental stability. Managing stress, therefore, means stabilizing Vata through regular routine, adequate rest, proper digestion, emotional balance, and timely recovery. By addressing stress at this functional level, Ayurveda aims to prevent the progression from reversible imbalance to irreversible disease.

6.5 Types of Stress Loads in the Human Machine

Stress is not a single uniform force acting on the human body. Just as machines experience different types of loads—thermal, mechanical, electrical, and chemical—the human body is subjected to multiple forms of stress, each affecting the system in a distinct way. These stress loads often act simultaneously and compound one another, gradually pushing the body beyond its adaptive capacity. Understanding these different stress loads helps explain why modern diseases are complex, multi-factorial, and progressive rather than sudden or isolated.

Psychological stress is one of the most common and least visible forms of load. It arises from work pressure, job insecurity, financial worries, relationship conflicts, social expectations, and constant mental stimulation from digital devices. A person may appear physically comfortable, sitting in an air-conditioned office or at home, yet the nervous system behaves as if facing a threat. The brain remains alert, thoughts race, and stress hormones circulate continuously. Over time, this constant mental tension leads to anxiety, depression, panic attacks, migraines, and functional digestive disorders such as irritable bowel syndrome. A simple example is an employee who lies awake at night replaying office problems in the mind; although the body is resting, the brain never switches off, slowly exhausting the nervous system.

Metabolic stress results from habits that disturb the body's energy balance. Irregular meals, excessive consumption of junk food and refined sugar, late-night eating, frequent snacking, and chronic sleep deprivation overload the metabolic machinery. The digestive system struggles to process inconsistent fuel, while hormones that regulate blood sugar and fat storage become imbalanced. Organs such as the liver, pancreas, and ovaries silently bear this load. Initially, the person may feel only fatigue or weight gain, but over time, metabolic diseases such as diabetes, fatty liver disease, polycystic ovarian syndrome, obesity, and chronic low energy develop. This is similar to feeding poor-quality fuel to an engine; it may run for some time, but efficiency drops and internal damage accumulates.

Inflammatory stress develops when the immune system is persistently activated. Chronic infections, autoimmune tendencies, environmental pollution, chemical exposure, poor gut health, and highly processed foods keep the immune system in a state of constant alert. Instead of attacking only harmful agents, the immune response begins to damage healthy tissues. This leads to diseases such as rheumatoid arthritis, systemic lupus erythematosus, psoriasis, and inflammatory bowel disease. From an engineering perspective, this is similar to corrosion in machinery. Rust does not cause immediate failure, but it slowly weakens structures from within until they become fragile and unreliable.

Mechanical stress arises from improper use of the body's structural framework. Poor posture, prolonged sitting, lack of regular movement, repetitive strain, and sudden overuse place uneven load on muscles, joints, and the spine. Just as misaligned machine parts wear out faster, improper body mechanics accelerate the degeneration of discs, cartilage, and joints. Over time, this results in cervical spondylosis, lumbar disc disease, knee osteoarthritis, shoulder stiffness, and chronic back pain. A common example is prolonged mobile phone use with a bent neck, which gradually leads to neck pain and nerve compression without any obvious injury.

These different stress loads rarely occur in isolation. Psychological stress often leads to poor eating habits and sleep deprivation, increasing metabolic stress. Metabolic imbalance promotes inflammation, which further weakens tissues and increases pain. Mechanical stress worsens when muscles are fatigued and poorly nourished. Thus, stress loads interact and amplify one another, creating a cycle of overload. This explains why many individuals suffer from multiple complaints at the same time—such as back pain, digestive issues, fatigue, and anxiety—rather than a single disease.

A simple everyday example illustrates this interaction. Consider a person working long hours at a desk job. Mental deadlines create psychological stress. Skipped meals and fast food cause metabolic stress. Poor posture creates mechanical stress. Lack of sleep and poor diet increase inflammation.

Initially, the person experiences minor discomforts, but over the years, these stresses accumulate and manifest as chronic illness. The body does not fail suddenly; it gradually gives way under multiple, unrelieved loads.

Recognizing stress as a combination of different loads shifts the focus from treating isolated symptoms to managing total system burden. Just as engineers assess all forces acting on a structure before designing solutions, maintaining human health requires understanding and reducing psychological, metabolic, inflammatory, and mechanical stress together. Only then can the human machine operate efficiently, sustainably, and without premature breakdown.

6.6 Stress Load Curve: Engineering vs the Human Body

In engineering, the behavior of materials under load follows a well-defined pattern known as the stress–strain curve. When a material is subjected to force within its elastic limit, it temporarily changes shape but returns to its original form once the load is removed. This phase is considered safe and reversible. However, when the load exceeds this elastic zone, the material enters the plastic zone, where deformation becomes permanent. Even if the load is reduced, the original shape is not fully restored. Beyond this lies the failure zone, where cracks propagate rapidly, and structural collapse occurs. Engineers use this understanding to design safety margins and plan maintenance long before visible damage appears.

The human body follows a remarkably similar stress load curve, although the process is biological rather than mechanical. In the initial adaptive phase, the body responds to stress by mobilizing internal reserves. Energy stores are used, stress hormones rise, and performance may even improve temporarily. A person under pressure may work longer hours, think faster, and appear highly productive. This phase gives the illusion that the body is coping well, just as a metal spring stretches without breaking under moderate load. However, this adaptability has limits and depends on adequate recovery.

When stress continues without sufficient rest, the body enters the exhaustion phase. In this stage, early warning symptoms begin to appear.

Sleep becomes disturbed, digestion becomes irregular, energy levels fluctuate, mood becomes unstable, and minor aches and pains become frequent. These symptoms are often ignored or suppressed with stimulants, painkillers, or temporary fixes. This stage is equivalent to the plastic zone in engineering, where damage has begun but collapse has not yet occurred. The body can no longer fully restore balance even when stress is briefly reduced.

If overload persists, the body progresses into the breakdown phase. At this point, structural and functional damage becomes established, and disease manifests clearly. Hypertension, diabetes, heart disease, autoimmune disorders, depression, and degenerative joint conditions emerge. This is the biological equivalent of material failure, where the structure can no longer support load. Recovery becomes difficult, expensive, and often incomplete, requiring long-term treatment rather than simple correction.

A common example helps illustrate this curve. Consider a rubber band. When stretched gently, it returns to its original shape. If stretched repeatedly beyond its limit, it loses elasticity. Eventually, one day it snaps. The snapping appears sudden, but the damage occurred gradually over time. Similarly, a person may tolerate long working hours, emotional strain, and poor lifestyle habits for years. When disease finally appears, it seems sudden, but the breakdown has been developing silently through the adaptive and exhaustion phases.

Most patients seek medical help only during the breakdown phase, when symptoms become severe enough to interfere with daily life. By this time, years of accumulated damage have already occurred. From an engineering perspective, this is equivalent to calling a technician only after a machine has completely failed, rather than servicing it when early warning signs appeared. Preventive maintenance is always cheaper, safer, and more effective than emergency repair.

Understanding the stress load curve emphasizes the importance of early intervention. Health protection should begin during the adaptive phase by ensuring adequate rest, nutrition, and recovery. During the exhaustion phase, timely correction can still reverse many changes. Once the breakdown phase is reached, treatment becomes complex and long-term. Just as engineers respect load limits to prevent structural failure, maintaining health requires respecting the body's adaptive capacity and acting before irreversible collapse occurs.

6.7 Clinical Case Examples

Clinical cases clearly demonstrate how chronic stress operates as a continuous mechanical load on the human system, leading to disease even in young and otherwise healthy individuals. A common example is that of a young executive with hypertension. Such an individual often appears physically fit and active, yet works long hours under constant deadlines, relies heavily on caffeine to maintain alertness, skips regular exercise, and sleeps poorly. His blood pressure rises not because of aging or genetic destiny, but because his cardiovascular system is functioning under a persistent high load without adequate recovery. From an engineering viewpoint, this resembles a pressure pipeline that is constantly kept at high pressure without scheduled shutdowns, eventually weakening the system. Ayurveda explains this condition as aggravation of Vata and Pitta along with depletion of Ojas, the body's protective and stabilizing energy, making the system vulnerable to breakdown.

Another clinically relevant example is autoimmune thyroid disease, which often develops after prolonged emotional stress, irregular meals, and chronic sleep deprivation. In such individuals, stress continuously disrupts digestion and metabolism, leading to the accumulation of metabolic waste. Over time, this waste interferes with immune regulation, causing the immune system to lose its ability to distinguish self from non-self. As a result, the immune system begins attacking the thyroid gland. In simple terms, this is similar to a misprogrammed security system that mistakenly identifies its own building as a threat and initiates damage from within. Ayurveda describes this process as disturbed Agni leading to Ama formation and subsequent involvement of deeper tissues, ultimately manifesting as autoimmune disease.

A third example can be seen in individuals suffering from chronic digestive disorders such as irritable bowel syndrome. These patients often have a long history of mental strain, irregular eating schedules, and constant worry. Initially, stress alters nerve signals to the gut, leading to irregular bowel movements, bloating, and abdominal discomfort. Over time, repeated stress keeps the digestive system in a hyper-responsive state, making symptoms persistent. From an engineering perspective, this resembles a control valve receiving erratic signals, causing irregular flow despite intact structural components. Ayurveda interprets this condition as a Vata disturbance affecting digestion and intestinal movement, rather than a structural disease of the gut.

Another common case involves stress-related diabetes in middle-aged individuals. Years of mental pressure, poor sleep, and irregular eating lead to repeated stress hormone release, raising blood sugar levels. Initially, the body compensates by increasing insulin production, but continuous overload exhausts this mechanism. Diabetes then becomes evident. This is similar to an engine running continuously at high speed; fuel consumption increases, efficiency drops, and components wear out prematurely. Ayurveda explains this progression through disturbed Agni, impaired tissue nourishment, and gradual depletion of metabolic balance.

These clinical examples highlight a critical insight: stress-related diseases do not arise from a single event or sudden failure. They develop gradually as a result of continuous overload on regulatory systems. The organs affected may differ, but the underlying mechanism remains the same—prolonged stress without recovery. Understanding disease through these real-life examples reinforces the importance of early stress management, adequate rest, and lifestyle correction. Just as engineers prevent system failure by managing load and ensuring downtime, human health depends on recognizing and reducing stress before irreversible damage occurs.

6.8 Stress and Hormonal Derailment

Hormones act as the body's internal communication signals, coordinating the activities of different organs much like messages transmitted through a control network. Under normal conditions, these signals are released in precise amounts and at specific times, maintaining balance in growth, metabolism, reproduction, and repair. Chronic stress disrupts this finely tuned communication system. When the body remains under constant stress, stress hormones dominate the hormonal environment, gradually distorting the timing, quantity, and sensitivity of other hormones. This derailment often begins silently, long before abnormalities appear in routine laboratory tests.

One of the earliest hormonal changes under chronic stress involves cortisol, the primary stress hormone. Normally, cortisol follows a daily rhythm—high in the morning to promote alertness and low at night to allow rest and repair. Persistent stress flattens or distorts this rhythm. Cortisol may remain elevated throughout the day or spike at inappropriate times. This continuous cortisol exposure interferes with sleep, raises blood sugar levels, and suppresses tissue repair. A simple example is a factory siren that is meant to sound only during emergencies; if it rings all day, workers become confused, exhausted, and inefficient.

Stress also significantly affects thyroid function. The thyroid gland regulates metabolic speed and energy use. Under chronic stress, the brain reduces signals to the thyroid as a protective measure, conserving energy for perceived survival. As a result, thyroid activity may slow down or fluctuate, leading to symptoms such as fatigue, weight gain, cold intolerance, hair loss, and mental fog. Importantly, these symptoms may appear even when thyroid blood tests remain within "normal" ranges. This explains why many stressed individuals feel hypothyroid despite acceptable laboratory values. It is similar to an engine whose control system reduces speed to prevent overheating, even though the fuel supply appears normal.

Insulin regulation is another major casualty of chronic stress. Stress hormones raise blood sugar to provide quick energy during emergencies. When stress becomes continuous, blood sugar remains persistently elevated, forcing the pancreas to produce more insulin. Over time, body cells become less responsive to insulin, a condition known as insulin resistance. This sets the stage for diabetes, weight gain, and metabolic syndrome. A common example is a person who experiences constant work pressure and relies on sugary snacks or caffeine for energy. Initially, this seems helpful, but gradually, energy crashes become frequent, and metabolic health declines.

Sex hormones are particularly sensitive to stress. In women, chronic stress disrupts the balance of estrogen, progesterone, and ovulatory signals, leading to conditions such as polycystic ovarian syndrome, irregular menstrual cycles, infertility, and worsening premenstrual symptoms. In men, stress reduces testosterone levels, contributing to erectile dysfunction, reduced sperm quality, fatigue, and low motivation. From a biological perspective, the body prioritizes survival over reproduction during prolonged stress. A simple analogy is a household cutting expenses on non-essential activities during a financial crisis; reproductive functions are downregulated to conserve resources.

Stress-related hormonal imbalance often develops before overt disease becomes evident. Many individuals experience unexplained infertility, irregular cycles, or sexual dysfunction despite normal scans and blood reports. This is because stress affects hormone receptors, timing, and tissue response, not just hormone levels themselves. Just as a mobile network may fail due to poor signal reception despite functional towers, hormonal communication may fail despite normal hormone production.

Another important aspect is the interaction between hormones. Cortisol interferes with thyroid hormone conversion, worsens insulin resistance, and suppresses sex hormone production. This interconnected disruption explains why stressed individuals often suffer from multiple hormonal issues simultaneously. Treating one hormone in isolation often provides limited relief because the underlying stress load remains unaddressed.

In practical terms, stress silently hijacks the endocrine system by shifting the body into a constant survival mode. Hormonal harmony, which requires rhythm, rest, and recovery, is lost. The consequences appear gradually as fatigue, weight changes, reproductive issues, mood disturbances, and metabolic disease. Understanding stress as the root cause of hormonal derailment highlights the importance of restoring balance through adequate sleep, mental calm, proper nutrition, and recovery—rather than relying solely on hormone replacement or symptomatic treatment.

6.9 Why Stress Causes Multi-Organ Disease

Stress rarely damages a single organ because it does not act at the level of individual parts; it acts at the level of control and coordination. In the human body, systems such as the nervous system, hormonal network, and immune regulation function like a central command unit. When stress activates this command unit continuously, it alters how every organ receives instructions. Cellular signaling becomes distorted, timing between systems is lost, and the body's ability to coordinate complex functions declines. As a result, disease does not remain confined to one location but gradually involves multiple organs and systems simultaneously.

One of the primary ways stress causes widespread disease is by altering cellular signaling. Cells communicate using chemical messengers and electrical signals that tell them when to grow, repair, rest, or defend. Chronic stress floods the body with stress hormones that override normal signaling. Cells remain in a defensive or emergency state instead of a repair state. Over time, this leads to poor healing, abnormal growth, and functional exhaustion. A simple example is a factory where the emergency alarm keeps ringing; workers stop normal production and focus only on survival tasks, leading to an overall decline in output and quality.

Stress also damages mitochondria, the energy-producing units of cells. Under continuous stress, energy production becomes inefficient, and cells shift from efficient fuel use to survival mode. This results in fatigue, muscle weakness, brain fog, and reduced organ performance. Because every organ depends on energy, mitochondrial dysfunction affects the entire body rather than a single organ. This is similar to a power plant producing unstable electricity; lights may flicker in every building rather than one specific location going dark.

Another critical effect of stress is the reduction of repair and regeneration mechanisms. Normally, the body constantly repairs tissues, replaces damaged cells, and maintains balance. Chronic stress suppresses these processes to conserve energy for perceived threats. As a result, wear and tear accumulate faster than repair. Joints degenerate, blood vessels stiffen, nerves lose insulation, and organs become less resilient. A common example is a road that develops potholes faster than they can be repaired; eventually, the entire road network deteriorates, not just one stretch.

Stress also weakens coordination between systems. The nervous system, endocrine system, immune system, and digestive system must work in harmony for health. Chronic stress disrupts this coordination. Hormonal rhythms become irregular, immune responses become exaggerated or suppressed, digestion becomes inefficient, and circulation becomes erratic. This explains why a stressed person may simultaneously suffer from digestive problems, skin disorders, joint pain, fatigue, and mood disturbances. The issue is not multiple unrelated diseases but one underlying control failure.

A simple everyday example illustrates this clearly. Consider a smartphone with a faulty operating system. Multiple apps begin to malfunction at once—battery drains quickly, calls drop, screen freezes, and performance slows. Replacing individual apps does not solve the problem because the root issue lies in the operating system. Similarly, stress disrupts the body's operating system. Treating one organ without correcting stress often leads to partial or temporary improvement, followed by new symptoms elsewhere.

Because stress acts systemically, its effects accumulate over time. Initially, the body compensates by diverting resources and suppressing symptoms. Over the years, these compensations fail, and multi-organ disease becomes evident. Conditions such as metabolic syndrome, autoimmune disorders, chronic pain syndromes, depression with physical illness, and accelerated aging are classic examples of stress-induced systemic failure.

Understanding stress as a central control disruptor explains why modern diseases are complex and interconnected. The solution, therefore, lies not in chasing individual symptoms but in restoring coordination, reducing stress load, and supporting cellular repair. Just as engineers fix a malfunctioning control unit rather than replacing every damaged machine, restoring health requires addressing stress at the system level to prevent widespread breakdown.

6.10 Stress Load Management: The Engineering Solution

In engineering, the longevity of any machine depends not on how powerful it is, but on how intelligently its load is managed. Machines are protected through load balancing, scheduled downtime, proper lubrication, and periodic overhaul. Continuous operation without rest, even at moderate load, leads to overheating, wear, and premature failure. The human body follows the same principle, but its maintenance protocols are biological rather than mechanical. Stress load management in humans is therefore not a luxury; it is a fundamental requirement for long-term function and survival.

Sleep is the most critical form of scheduled downtime for the human system. During sleep, the nervous system resets, stress hormones decline, tissues repair, memory consolidates, and metabolic waste is cleared from the brain. When sleep is inadequate or irregular, the body loses its primary recovery window. A simple example is a factory that never shuts down for maintenance; machines continue running, but internal damage accumulates until a sudden breakdown occurs. Similarly, chronic sleep deprivation forces the body to operate continuously in stress mode, accelerating disease development.

Nutrition functions as fuel quality control. Just as machines require clean, compatible fuel to function efficiently, the human body requires regular, wholesome, and digestible food. Under stress, people often rely on fast food, excess sugar, caffeine, or irregular meals, which further overload digestion and metabolism. Proper nutrition supports stable blood sugar, balanced hormones, and efficient energy production. For example, an engine running on contaminated fuel may still run, but carbon buildup and inefficiency develop. Likewise, poor dietary choices under stress worsen fatigue, inflammation, and metabolic imbalance.

Detoxification represents waste removal and system cleaning. In machines, accumulated sludge, carbon deposits, and debris reduce efficiency and increase friction. Periodic cleaning restores performance. In the human body, stress impairs digestion and elimination, leading to the accumulation of metabolic waste. Natural detoxification through proper digestion, hydration, sweating, and elimination reduces this burden. Ayurveda emphasizes supporting the body's natural cleaning mechanisms rather than aggressive intervention. A simple example is cleaning household water pipes; regular maintenance prevents blockage and pressure damage.

Mind regulation is the biological equivalent of load redistribution. In engineering, excessive load on one component is redistributed to prevent failure. In humans, unregulated mental stress concentrates load on the nervous and hormonal systems. Practices that calm the mind, regulate breathing, and improve emotional resilience redistribute this load, allowing systems to recover. For instance, taking short breaks during intense work prevents mental overheating, much like cooling fans prevent engine damage.

Ayurveda translates these engineering principles into practical daily and seasonal routines. Daily routines stabilize biological rhythms, ensuring regular sleep, meals, and activity. Seasonal adaptation adjusts diet and lifestyle to environmental changes, preventing additional stress. Oil massage acts as biological lubrication, calming the nervous system, improving circulation, and reducing muscular tension. Therapies that stabilize brain function help reset stress circuits and promote deep relaxation. These practices are not rituals or beliefs; they are maintenance protocols designed to preserve system integrity.

A simple everyday example illustrates this approach. A person working long hours who adopts regular sleep, balanced meals, brief relaxation breaks, and periodic rest finds energy returning and symptoms reducing. Without these measures, medication alone provides only temporary relief. Just as machines last longer with regular servicing than emergency repairs, the human body thrives when stress load is managed proactively.

Ultimately, stress load management is preventive engineering applied to human health. It focuses on maintaining balance, preventing overload, and ensuring timely recovery. By respecting biological design limits and applying maintenance principles consistently, disease progression can be slowed, halted, or even reversed before irreversible breakdown occurs.

6.11 Key Insight

Stress rarely causes sudden death or immediate illness. Instead, it acts slowly, quietly, and cumulatively, producing what can be best described as a gradual mechanical failure of the human system. Just as machines do not break down in a single moment without warning, the human body does not suddenly become diseased without a long period of overload. Chronic stress continuously strains the body's control systems—nervous, hormonal, metabolic, and immune—weakening them little by little. The final disease that appears is not the beginning of the problem; it is the visible endpoint of prolonged internal deterioration.

A chronically stressed body often appears functional for years. People continue to work, raise families, and fulfill responsibilities despite poor sleep, irregular meals, emotional strain, and constant mental pressure. This outward functionality creates a false sense of security. The situation is similar to a cracked bridge that continues to carry traffic daily. Vehicles pass without incident, and the structure seems safe. However, each passing load widens the cracks and weakens the internal framework. When collapse finally occurs, it appears sudden, but the damage was present long before the event.

This understanding explains why many serious illnesses are diagnosed unexpectedly. A person may feel "normal" until the day blood pressure readings become dangerously high, blood sugar crosses diagnostic limits, or a heart attack occurs. These events seem abrupt, yet they are the result of years of accumulated stress load. Just as rust weakens steel silently, stress weakens tissues, vessels, nerves, and organs without causing immediate pain. By the time symptoms force attention, the system has already lost much of its reserve capacity.

Preventing disease, therefore, is not about fear or constant medical testing. It is about respecting the design limits of the human body. Every system has a tolerance for load, beyond which damage begins. Continuous overwork, chronic emotional strain, lack of sleep, poor nutrition, and absence of recovery are forms of misuse, not bad luck. A simple example is a motorbike ridden at high speed every day without servicing. It may run well initially, but engine life shortens dramatically. Regular maintenance, not panic repairs, preserves performance.

Another everyday example can be seen in personal finances. Small, repeated expenses that exceed income may seem manageable day to day, but over time, they lead to debt and crisis. The crisis appears sudden, yet it was created by a prolonged imbalance. Similarly, stress-related disease is a result of long-term imbalance between load and recovery. The body keeps compensating until it no longer can.

Intelligent health maintenance focuses on early signs of overload—fatigue, poor sleep, digestive disturbance, irritability, reduced enthusiasm, and frequent minor illnesses. These are not trivial complaints; they are early warning indicators, much like unusual noise or vibration in a machine. Addressing them early prevents major breakdown later.

The key insight, therefore, is that health is preserved not by heroic interventions after collapse, but by consistent, intelligent maintenance before failure occurs. Respecting biological limits, allowing regular recovery, and managing stress proactively keep the human machine functional, resilient, and long-lasting. Disease prevention is not fear-driven medicine; it is applied engineering wisdom for human life.

Chapter 7

Repair & Regeneration Engineering

How the Human Body Fixes Itself—and Why It Sometimes Fails

7.1 Repair Is Not an Emergency Process—It Is a Continuous Engineering Function

In engineering, the idea of repair is inseparable from the idea of design itself. No engineer ever assumes that a machine will run forever without wear. From the moment a machine starts operating, forces such as friction, heat, vibration, pressure, and chemical reactions begin to act on its components. A car engine slowly wears down at the piston rings, a bridge develops micro-cracks due to repeated load, and even a smartphone processor degrades due to heat generated during daily use. Because this damage is expected, engineers do not wait for breakdowns. They design lubrication systems to reduce friction, cooling systems to remove excess heat, sensors to detect early faults, and maintenance schedules to restore performance before failure occurs. Machines fail not because damage occurs, but because maintenance is delayed or ignored.

The human body operates on exactly the same principle, but with far greater intelligence and automation. Unlike machines that require external technicians, the body performs its own inspection, diagnosis, and repair every moment of life. With every breath we take, oxygen produces energy but also generates free radicals that can damage cells. With every meal, digestion creates nutrients but also metabolic waste. With every step, muscle contraction creates strength but also microscopic tears. Even thinking and emotional stress place a measurable load on the nervous system. If such damage were not constantly repaired, the body would collapse within hours. Health exists because the body is continuously correcting these small injuries without our conscious awareness.

At the microscopic level, this repair work is astonishingly precise. DNA strands, which store genetic information, are damaged thousands of times daily due to normal metabolism and environmental exposure. Specialized repair enzymes immediately locate and fix these breaks, much like a spell-check system correcting errors in a document as it is typed. Proteins that lose their functional shape due to heat or stress are either refolded or dismantled and rebuilt. Cells that are too damaged to function safely are instructed to self-destruct in an orderly manner, preventing harm to surrounding tissues. This silent, background activity is the true reason why the body appears stable despite continuous internal chaos.

A useful layman's example is that of a well-managed city. Roads develop small potholes every day due to traffic and weather. Garbage is generated daily by households. Electrical lines face minor faults due to load fluctuations. A city remains livable not because these problems do not occur, but because repair crews work continuously, often at night, before citizens even notice. If garbage collection stops, waste piles up. If road repairs are delayed, accidents increase. If electrical maintenance is ignored, blackouts occur. Similarly, the body's internal "maintenance departments" work nonstop to keep tissues functional and safe.

Disease, therefore, should not be viewed as the sudden arrival of damage, but as the gradual failure of repair systems. For example, everyone experiences minor joint cartilage damage daily while walking, but joints remain healthy as long as repair keeps pace with wear. Everyone experiences brief spikes in blood sugar after meals, but diabetes develops only when metabolic repair and regulation fail over time. Everyone is exposed to stress hormones, but mental illness or hypertension develops only when recovery mechanisms such as sleep, relaxation, and hormonal reset are repeatedly denied. The damage was always present; the difference lies in the body's ability to recover.

An everyday analogy is rust on metal. A small amount of rust forms quickly when metal is exposed to moisture, but if the metal is regularly cleaned, painted, and protected, it lasts for decades. If maintenance is ignored, rust spreads silently underneath until the structure suddenly collapses. The collapse appears sudden, but the failure was long in the making. In the same way, symptoms such as pain, ulcers, fatigue, or organ failure appear late. By the time they are noticed, repair failure has already been progressing for years.

Understanding repair as a continuous process changes how health and medicine are perceived. Treatment should not be limited to emergency symptom control, just as engineering does not rely only on breakdown repairs. True healthcare focuses on strengthening daily repair capacity through proper nutrition, adequate rest, stress regulation, efficient digestion, and timely detoxification. When repair systems are supported, the body can tolerate enormous stress and still return to balance. When repair systems are neglected, even small stresses become dangerous. Thus, health is not the absence of damage, but the uninterrupted success of repair.

7.2 Damage Is Inevitable; Failure Is Optional

In both engineering and biology, damage is not a sign of failure; it is a normal consequence of use. Any system that functions continuously must accept wear as part of its operation. Modern medicine often intervenes only when damage becomes obvious—when pain appears, swelling restricts movement, ulcers bleed, or an organ begins to malfunction. At this stage, attention is focused on controlling symptoms or replacing failed parts. Ayurveda, by contrast, works on a more preventive engineering principle: if repair mechanisms are continuously supported, damage never reaches a level where it becomes visible or dangerous. Health is therefore not defined by the absence of stress or wear, but by the uninterrupted ability to self-correct.

Classical Ayurveda defines health as a condition in which body tissues remain balanced, nourished, and functionally stable. This concept is clearly stated in Charaka Samhita, where the equilibrium of tissues is described as the foundation of health. In simple terms, this means that minor disturbances are constantly neutralized before they grow into disease. Just as a well-designed machine absorbs vibration without breaking, a healthy body absorbs daily insults—poor sleep, emotional stress, minor infections, or dietary errors—without collapsing.

A common household example makes this principle easy to understand. Consider a house that develops small cracks in its walls due to seasonal temperature changes. These cracks are not unusual and do not immediately threaten the structure. If the owner inspects the house regularly and fills the cracks, the building remains strong for decades. However, if the cracks are ignored, rainwater enters, moisture corrodes steel reinforcements, and the foundation slowly weakens. One day, a wall suddenly collapses. To an outsider, the collapse looks sudden, but in reality, the failure was the result of years of neglected repair. The same logic applies to the human body.

The body continuously sends early warning signals long before disease becomes obvious. Persistent fatigue is a sign that energy repair is inadequate. Poor sleep indicates failure of nervous system recovery. Frequent infections suggest weakened immune repair. Slow wound healing points toward compromised tissue regeneration. These signs are comparable to warning lights on a machine dashboard. Ignoring them does not stop the damage; it only allows repair failure to deepen. By the time a clear diagnosis, such as diabetes, arthritis, or heart disease, is made, the imbalance has usually existed for many years.

Another simple example is eyesight. Almost everyone experiences eye strain from prolonged screen use. In a healthy system, rest, blinking, and tear production restore balance. If strain is continuous and recovery is denied, headaches, dryness, and vision problems develop. The damage was not sudden; the failure occurred because repair time was not provided. Similarly, joints experience daily micro-damage during walking and lifting.

When lubrication, nutrition, and rest are adequate, joints remain healthy. When these supports are missing, degeneration begins.

This understanding reframes disease not as bad luck or sudden attack, but as a predictable outcome of neglected maintenance. From an Ayurvedic perspective, lifestyle errors such as irregular eating, chronic stress, poor sleep, and suppression of natural urges slowly weaken repair intelligence. The body continues to function outwardly, just as a damaged bridge continues to carry traffic, but its safety margin steadily shrinks. Eventually, even a small additional stress causes visible failure.

Therefore, failure is optional, not because damage can be avoided, but because repair can be strengthened. When daily routines support digestion, sleep, mental calm, circulation, and tissue nourishment, the body remains resilient despite constant wear. When these supports are ignored, even normal life stresses become destructive. True medicine, like good engineering, does not wait for collapse. It maintains balance continuously so that damage never progresses into disease.

7.3 Multilayer Repair Engineering in the Human Body

Repair in the human body does not occur at a single point or in a single manner; it operates simultaneously at multiple interconnected levels, much like a well-managed city that maintains its roads, water pipelines, electricity grids, sewage systems, and communication networks all at once. If only roads are repaired, but water pipelines leak, the city still suffers. In the same way, true health exists only when repair functions smoothly at the molecular, cellular, tissue, and systemic levels together. Failure at any one level eventually affects all others, leading to disease.

At the **molecular level**, repair is extremely rapid and constant. Every cell in the body contains DNA, which acts as the instruction manual for life. Daily exposure to sunlight, air pollution, radiation, food metabolism, and even normal breathing causes tiny injuries to DNA and proteins. These injuries are unavoidable and occur thousands of times per cell per day. The body is equipped with specialized enzymes that scan DNA continuously, detect errors, and correct them immediately, much like software that automatically corrects spelling mistakes while typing. Alongside this, antioxidant systems neutralize toxic byproducts of metabolism, similar to how exhaust filters prevent smoke from damaging an engine. When these molecular repair systems weaken due to aging, poor nutrition, chronic stress, or toxin exposure, errors accumulate. Over time, this accumulation manifests as premature aging, cancer, autoimmune disorders, and unexplained inflammatory conditions.

At the **cellular level**, repair works through intelligent recycling and replacement. Cells are not meant to live forever; old or damaged cells are systematically dismantled through a process called autophagy. This process functions like a waste-recycling plant, where broken machinery is taken apart and reusable materials are salvaged to build new equipment. Autophagy keeps cells clean, efficient, and functional. Stem cells act as a reserve workforce, stepping in when specialized cells are lost due to injury or wear. For example, skin renews itself regularly, and blood cells are constantly replaced. When cellular repair slows down, damaged cells remain active instead of being removed. This leads to insulin resistance in diabetes, plaque buildup in arteries, and accumulation of toxic proteins in brain diseases. The problem is not excess damage, but poor recycling.

At the **tissue level**, repair becomes visible and follows a well-defined sequence. When tissue is injured, the body first initiates inflammation, which acts like a cleanup crew removing debris, dead cells, and microbes. Next comes the growth phase, where new cells, blood vessels, and connective tissue are formed to rebuild the damaged area. Finally, remodeling reshapes and strengthens the tissue so it can withstand normal load again. This process is similar to repairing a damaged road: debris is cleared, fresh material is laid, and the surface is compacted for durability. If inflammation lasts too long due to infection, poor circulation, or metabolic imbalance, repair stalls. If nutrition is inadequate, the rebuilt tissue is weak. This leads to chronic wounds, excessive scarring, fibrosis, or fragile tissues that break down repeatedly.

At the **systemic level**, repair is coordinated by the nervous system, hormones, and immune system working together. The nervous system decides whether the body is in a state of activity or recovery. Hormones act as managers, directing energy toward growth, repair, or conservation depending on age, time of day, and stress levels. The immune system performs dual roles: it cleans damaged tissue and protects against infection, while also ensuring that repair does not become excessive. When systemic coordination is healthy, repair happens efficiently during rest, especially during sleep. When this coordination fails, repair becomes chaotic. The immune system may attack healthy tissues, leading to autoimmune disease. Hormonal imbalance may prevent proper healing. The nervous system may remain stuck in a stress state, blocking recovery and causing chronic fatigue.

A simple daily-life example illustrates this integration clearly. After a minor cut on the skin, molecular repair seals damaged DNA, cellular repair removes dead cells, tissue repair closes the wound, and systemic repair ensures blood clotting, immune protection, and later scar remodeling. If even one level is compromised—such as poor blood sugar control, sleep deprivation, or chronic stress—the wound heals slowly or becomes infected. The cut itself is minor, but the repair environment is faulty.

Thus, multilayer repair engineering explains why the same injury heals quickly in one person but becomes chronic in another. Health is not determined by how much damage occurs, but by how effectively repair systems function at every level simultaneously. Strengthening only one layer while neglecting others produces incomplete healing. True regeneration requires harmony across molecular accuracy, cellular recycling, tissue rebuilding, and systemic coordination.

7.4 Repair Engineering in Ayurveda: Dhātu Poshana and Rasayana

Ayurveda understands repair not as a reaction to injury or disease, but as a continuous, lifelong process of nourishment and renewal. According to Ayurvedic physiology, the human body is sustained by seven fundamental tissues, called Dhātus, which are formed one after another in a precise sequence. Each Dhātu depends on the quality of the previous one, just as each stage of manufacturing depends on the quality of raw material supplied to it. If this chain of nourishment is uninterrupted and efficient, tissues remain strong, adaptable, and capable of self-repair. If the chain is disturbed, degeneration begins quietly, long before disease becomes visible.

The foundation of this repair system is digestion and metabolism. Ayurveda places great emphasis on Agni, the digestive and metabolic fire, because it determines how well food is converted into usable tissue nutrition. Even the most nutritious food is useless if digestion is weak, irregular, or overloaded. This can be compared to pouring premium fuel into an engine with a damaged combustion system—the fuel is present, but performance remains poor. In the body, weak digestion leads to poorly formed tissues, reduced repair capacity, and accumulation of metabolic waste, which blocks regeneration pathways.

Dhātu Poshana, or tissue nourishment, is not simply about eating more or taking supplements. It is about ensuring that nutrition reaches the right tissue, at the right time, in the right form. For example, muscles require adequate protein and circulation, bones require mineralization and stability, and nervous tissue requires fats and calm metabolic conditions. Ayurveda recognizes that stress, poor sleep, and improper routines can divert nutrition away from repair toward mere survival. As a result, tissues may exist but remain undernourished and fragile, leading to weakness, pain, or degeneration despite adequate food intake.

Rasayana therapy represents the highest level of Ayurvedic repair engineering. Rather than targeting a single symptom or organ, Rasayana strengthens the body's overall repair intelligence. It improves the quality of digestion, enhances circulation at the micro-level, supports immune balance, and stabilizes nervous system function. This holistic strengthening allows the body to repair damage more efficiently across all tissues. A simple analogy is updating the operating system of a machine so that all maintenance functions work better automatically, instead of repeatedly fixing individual faults as they arise.

In daily life, the effects of Rasayana can be easily understood. A person with good Rasayana support recovers faster from illness, heals wounds more quickly, tolerates stress better, and ages more slowly. Hair, skin, joints, digestion, and immunity all improve together, not because each problem is treated separately, but because the underlying repair environment is strengthened. In contrast, symptom-based treatment may temporarily reduce pain or inflammation but leaves the tissue weak and prone to repeated breakdown, similar to repeatedly patching a leak without fixing the faulty pipe.

Classical Ayurvedic texts, especially the Rasayana sections of Charaka Samhita, emphasize that Rasayana is meant not only for the sick but also for healthy individuals. This highlights an important engineering insight: repair capacity must be built before failure occurs. Just as preventive maintenance extends the life of machines, Rasayana preserves tissue quality, delays degeneration, and maintains resilience throughout life.

In summary, Ayurveda's approach to repair engineering is deeply preventive and systemic. Dhātu Poshana ensures that tissues are continuously nourished, while Rasayana strengthens the intelligence that governs repair, adaptation, and regeneration. Together, they transform the body from a fragile system that breaks under stress into a resilient system capable of absorbing damage and restoring balance naturally.

7.5 Clinical Example: Non-Healing Wound

A non-healing wound is one of the clearest real-life demonstrations of repair failure in the human body. In modern clinical practice, such wounds are usually explained using visible and measurable factors such as poor blood circulation, uncontrolled diabetes, persistent infection, pressure over the wound, or deficiency of collagen and proteins. These explanations are accurate but incomplete, because they describe *what is going wrong at the surface* without fully addressing *why the body's repair machinery is unable to correct it*. From an engineering perspective, these are signs of system malfunction rather than root causes.

Ayurveda approaches the same condition by evaluating the internal repair environment rather than the wound alone. It explains non-healing wounds as a result of impaired blood quality, blockage in microcirculation channels, weak digestive and metabolic power, and dominance of degenerative forces that dry, stiffen, or starve tissues. In simple terms, Ayurveda asks whether the body has the right materials, energy, circulation, and coordination to perform repair. If any of these are compromised, even a small wound can persist for months.

A simple farming analogy helps clarify this concept. Imagine a plant that is not growing well. Adding fertilizer alone may not help if the soil is hard, water cannot reach the roots, or sunlight is blocked. The problem is not the seed or the fertilizer, but the *environment*. Similarly, applying dressings or antibiotics to a wound may reduce infection temporarily, but healing will not progress unless the internal environment becomes supportive. The wound is like the plant leaf that shows damage, while the soil represents digestion, circulation, and metabolism.

Consider a common example of a diabetic foot ulcer. The wound itself may be small, but high blood sugar damages blood vessels, reduces oxygen delivery, and weakens immune response. At the same time, digestion may be impaired, leading to poor-quality tissue formation. Even if advanced dressings are applied, the wound struggles to heal because the body cannot supply healthy building material or coordinate repair. Once blood sugar is controlled, digestion improves, circulation is supported, and inflammation is balanced, the same wound often begins to heal steadily. This clearly shows that repair depends more on the internal system than on the wound size.

Another everyday example is a cut on the skin in two different individuals. In a healthy young person with good sleep, appetite, and circulation, a cut heals quickly with minimal scarring. In an elderly person with poor nutrition, anemia, stress, and chronic illness, the same cut may take weeks to close or become infected. The injury is identical, but the repair capacity is different. This demonstrates that non-healing wounds are not a local skin problem, but a whole-body repair issue.

Ayurveda emphasizes correcting digestion because all tissue repair depends on properly processed nutrition. If digestion is weak, the body produces poorly formed tissue, just as a construction site using low-quality cement produces weak walls. Blocked channels prevent nutrients and oxygen from reaching the wound, similar to blocked water pipes preventing irrigation. Degenerative forces dominate when tissues become dry, cold, or depleted, slowing cell division and collagen formation. Unless these underlying issues are corrected, repeated wound care becomes only a temporary solution.

From a repair engineering viewpoint, effective wound healing requires restoring the *repair ecosystem*. This includes clearing infection, ensuring adequate circulation, supplying proper nutrition, correcting digestion, reducing metabolic waste, and supporting immune balance. When this environment is restored, the body resumes its natural healing program, often with minimal external intervention. Thus, a non-healing wound is not merely a failure of skin repair, but a visible signal that the body's internal maintenance system needs comprehensive correction rather than isolated treatment.

7.6 Clinical Example: Degenerative Joint Disease

Degenerative joint disease provides a clear and easily understandable example of how repair failure develops slowly over time. From an engineering point of view, a joint functions much like a mechanical bearing that allows smooth movement between two surfaces. In machines, bearings are designed to handle load and reduce friction, but only when they are adequately lubricated and periodically serviced. If lubrication dries up or load becomes excessive, friction increases, heat is generated, surfaces begin to wear unevenly, and eventually the bearing produces noise, stiffness, and failure. The damage does not occur suddenly; it progresses silently over the years.

In the human body, joints are built on the same principle. Cartilage acts as a smooth, shock-absorbing surface, and synovial fluid provides lubrication and nutrition to this cartilage. With normal movement, joints experience micro-damage every day, but this damage is continuously repaired as long as nutrition, circulation, and lubrication are adequate. Degenerative joint disease begins when synovial fluid quality decreases, circulation to joint tissues becomes poor, and low-grade inflammation persists. As lubrication reduces, friction increases, leading to cartilage thinning, stiffness, and pain.

A common daily-life example is the door hinge in a house. When oiled regularly, the hinge moves silently for years. If oiling is neglected, the hinge starts making noise, becomes stiff, and eventually rusts or breaks. Applying force to move it may temporarily open the door, but the underlying damage continues. Similarly, painkillers may temporarily allow movement in arthritic joints, but they do not restore lubrication or repair cartilage. The warning sound is silenced, but the hinge continues to wear.

Ayurveda approaches joint degeneration as a failure of nourishment, lubrication, and nervous system coordination. Oil application therapies provide external lubrication and also improve local circulation, allowing nutrients to reach joint tissues. Medicated enemas, which act through the colon and nervous system, help regulate muscle tone, improve joint nutrition, and reduce degenerative forces. These therapies function like a comprehensive servicing process rather than a single repair action. They do not merely reduce pain but improve the internal conditions required for tissue regeneration.

Rasayana herbs play a crucial role in supporting deeper repair. They strengthen bone and marrow tissues, improve metabolic efficiency, and slow degeneration. This is comparable to replacing worn machine parts with higher-quality materials rather than simply adjusting the machine to work with damaged components. Over time, improved nourishment and metabolic support allow joints to regain some cushioning, flexibility, and strength, reducing the rate of further degeneration.

A practical clinical observation supports this concept. Two individuals with similar X-ray findings of joint degeneration may have very different symptoms and outcomes. One person, with good digestion, proper lubrication, and regular maintenance through lifestyle and therapy, may remain functional with minimal pain. Another person, with poor sleep, chronic stress, obesity, and inadequate nutrition, may deteriorate rapidly. The structural damage may appear similar, but the repair environment differs greatly.

This example highlights an important engineering insight: pain is not the disease; it is a warning signal. Suppressing pain without improving repair is equivalent to disabling an alarm system in a failing machine. True repair engineering aims to restore lubrication, reduce friction, improve nutrition, and rebalance load distribution. When these principles are applied consistently, joints may not become "new," but they can remain functional, stable, and pain-controlled for years. Degenerative joint disease, therefore, is not an inevitable consequence of aging, but often a reflection of neglected maintenance and impaired repair capacity.

7.7 Why Repair Fails: Common Engineering Errors

Repair failure in the human body follows predictable patterns, very similar to failures seen in engineering systems. Machines rarely fail because of a single large error; they fail because of repeated small mistakes that accumulate over time. One of the most common errors is continuous overload without adequate rest. In engineering, machines are designed with duty cycles that include active time and recovery time. Running a machine nonstop without a shutdown leads to overheating, metal fatigue, and early breakdown. In the human body, chronic stress, long working hours, constant mental stimulation, and inadequate sleep create the same effect. Cells require rest periods—especially during sleep—to repair DNA, recycle damaged components, and reset hormonal balance. When rest is denied, repair slows, damage accumulates, and fatigue, immunity loss, and chronic disease follow.

Another major error is poor-quality raw material. No engineer would expect a building to last if it is constructed with weak steel or inferior cement. Similarly, the human body cannot repair itself properly without adequate nutrition. Processed foods, excess sugar, unhealthy fats, and nutrient-poor diets deprive the body of essential building blocks such as proteins, minerals, and healthy fats. Even when calories are sufficient, the quality of nutrition may be inadequate. This leads to weak tissue repair, slow healing, fragile bones, and reduced immunity. The body may appear well-fed but remains structurally undernourished, much like a structure that looks complete but lacks internal strength.

A third critical reason for repair failure is blockage of repair pathways due to chronic inflammation. In engineering terms, even the best repair materials are useless if supply lines are blocked. Clogged pipes prevent water flow, jammed conveyors halt production, and corroded wiring disrupts communication. In the body, chronic low-grade inflammation blocks circulation, interferes with insulin signaling, and disrupts hormonal communication. This prevents nutrients and oxygen from reaching tissues that need repair. Conditions such as obesity, insulin resistance, autoimmune disorders, and long-standing infections create an internal environment where repair signals cannot reach their destination, even if the body has the capacity to heal.

Late intervention is another common and costly engineering error. Preventive maintenance is always cheaper and more effective than emergency repair. Once a bridge collapses, no amount of maintenance can restore it; it must be rebuilt. Similarly, when tissue damage progresses to irreversible structural loss—such as advanced cartilage destruction, extensive nerve damage, or organ fibrosis—repair becomes limited. Modern medicine often encounters patients at this late stage, where treatment focuses on managing symptoms rather than restoring structure. Ayurveda emphasizes early correction, when functional imbalance is still reversible and repair systems can be reactivated.

Ayurveda groups these errors under the concept of misuse of lifestyle and neglect of bodily intelligence. Excessive physical strain, irregular routines, improper diet, suppression of natural urges, and chronic mental stress are all viewed as violations of the body's design limits. The body continuously communicates its needs through hunger, fatigue, pain, and emotional signals. Ignoring these signals is comparable to ignoring warning alarms in a machine. The machine may continue to run for some time, but the cost of failure increases with every ignored alert.

A simple daily-life example ties these errors together. Consider a delivery vehicle used continuously without rest, fueled with poor-quality diesel, driven on damaged roads, and serviced only after breakdown. Such a vehicle will fail early despite being well-designed. In contrast, a vehicle used within limits, fueled properly, serviced regularly, and repaired early will last many years. The human body follows the same principles. Repair failure is not mysterious or random; it is the predictable outcome of overload, poor input, blocked pathways, and delayed correction.

Therefore, prevention is always easier than reconstruction. Supporting daily repair through proper sleep, nutrition, stress management, timely detoxification, and early intervention preserves health and resilience. Once repair systems are protected, the body can withstand damage without progressing to disease. Repair does not fail suddenly; it fails when engineering principles are repeatedly violated over time.

7.8 Regeneration Engineering: Integrating Modern Science and Ayurveda (Expanded Explanation)

True regeneration in the human body is not the result of a single medicine, procedure, or therapy; it is the outcome of multiple systems working in harmony. Just as restoring a damaged building requires proper materials, skilled labor, uninterrupted power, and correct timing, biological regeneration requires rest, adequate nutrition, efficient circulation, hormonal balance, immune intelligence, and mental calm. If even one of these elements is missing, repair becomes slow, incomplete, or faulty. Both modern science and Ayurveda recognize this truth, though they describe and approach it using different languages.

Modern biomedical science has clearly demonstrated the importance of **rest and sleep** in regeneration. During deep sleep, the brain clears metabolic waste, growth hormones are released, DNA repair accelerates, and immune memory is strengthened. This is comparable to shutting down a factory at night so that machines can be cleaned, recalibrated, and serviced. A person who sleeps well heals faster after injury, resists infection better, and ages more slowly than someone who is chronically sleep-deprived, regardless of medication use. Without rest, even the most advanced treatments produce limited results.

Nutrition and metabolic health form the next pillar of regeneration. Modern research on proteins, micronutrients, gut health, and insulin regulation shows that tissues cannot regenerate without proper building blocks and metabolic balance. Stem cell research has revealed that stem cells remain inactive or dysfunctional in hostile metabolic environments such as chronic inflammation or high blood sugar. This is similar to having skilled workers but no raw materials or a polluted worksite. Ayurveda emphasizes this same principle by insisting that food must be compatible, digestible, and suited to individual capacity so that nutrition is actually converted into tissue repair rather than waste.

Circulation and detoxification are equally critical. Modern medicine recognizes that oxygen delivery, blood flow, and lymphatic drainage are essential for healing. Poor circulation leads to slow wound healing, nerve damage, and organ dysfunction. Ayurveda describes this as blockage of channels, where nutrients and signals fail to reach tissues. Detoxification, whether through modern metabolic clearance or Ayurvedic cleansing methods, can be compared to clearing blocked roads so that repair crews can reach damaged sites. Without clearing waste, repair efforts are inefficient and short-lived.

Hormonal balance and immune intelligence act as master regulators of regeneration. Hormones decide whether the body is in growth mode, repair mode, or survival mode. Chronic stress keeps the body locked in survival mode, diverting energy away from regeneration. The immune system, meanwhile, must clean damaged tissue without attacking healthy structures. Modern science shows that immune dysregulation leads to autoimmunity or chronic inflammation, both of which block repair. Ayurveda similarly emphasizes balance, recognizing that excessive or deficient immune responses both impair healing. Regeneration requires intelligent regulation, not overreaction.

Ayurveda's contribution to regeneration engineering lies in its **holistic integration of lifestyle, time, and environment**. Daily routines, seasonal adaptation, mental discipline, and Rasayana therapy are designed to maintain repair readiness at all times. Rasayana does not merely target disease; it strengthens digestion, circulation, immunity, and mental stability together. This is similar to maintaining a machine in optimal condition so that breakdowns become rare rather than repeatedly fixing individual faults. Classical texts such as the Rasayana sections of Charaka Samhita emphasize that regeneration is a lifelong process, not a crisis response.

A simple example makes this integration clear. Imagine two houses exposed to the same weather. One is cleaned regularly, ventilated, repaired promptly, and maintained according to the season. The other is neglected until visible damage appears. When heavy rain arrives, the first house remains safe, while the second develops leaks and structural damage. Both faced the same stress, but their maintenance systems differed. Similarly, two individuals may face the same illness or injury, but the one with integrated regeneration practices recovers faster and more completely.

In conclusion, regeneration engineering is strongest when modern science and Ayurveda are combined rather than treated as opposing systems. Modern science explains the mechanisms of repair, while Ayurveda provides a practical framework for sustaining those mechanisms daily. Together, they shift medicine away from fragmented symptom control toward intelligent system maintenance. True healing occurs not when disease is suppressed, but when the body's innate capacity to repair, adapt, and renew is fully supported.

7.9 Key Takeaway: Repair Capacity Determines Health

The most important lesson from repair and regeneration engineering is that damage itself is not the true enemy of health. Damage is an unavoidable consequence of living, moving, thinking, and interacting with the environment. Every breath produces metabolic stress, every movement creates microscopic tissue strain, and every emotional response alters hormonal balance. The human body is designed with this reality in mind. It is built not to avoid damage, but to repair it continuously. Health exists as long as this repair capacity remains strong, responsive, and unobstructed. Disease begins when this capacity is ignored, exhausted, or blocked for long periods of time.

A simple engineering analogy makes this principle clear. Consider a commercial airplane. Engineers do not expect aircraft components to remain flawless forever. Instead, they design strict maintenance schedules that inspect, service, and replace parts long before failure occurs. An aircraft accident rarely happens because a part wore out unexpectedly; it happens because maintenance protocols were skipped or warning signs were ignored. In the same way, the human body rarely collapses suddenly without prior signals. Fatigue, disturbed sleep, poor digestion, reduced immunity, and slow healing are all signs that repair systems are under strain. When these signals are addressed early, breakdown can be prevented.

In everyday life, this concept can be seen in physical fitness. Muscles grow stronger not during exercise, but during rest and recovery after exercise. Exercise creates damage; rest allows repair. If exercise is excessive and recovery is inadequate, injury and weakness develop instead of strength. This shows that stress itself is not harmful—lack of recovery is. The same principle applies to mental work, emotional stress, and metabolic load. Continuous effort without recovery exhausts repair reserves, leading to burnout, chronic illness, and degeneration.

Medicine often focuses on fighting disease once it becomes visible, similar to repairing a machine only after it breaks down. While emergency intervention is sometimes necessary, it is not a sustainable model for long-term health. True healing occurs when the internal repair environment is restored so that the body can correct itself. Painkillers may reduce discomfort, antibiotics may control infection, and surgery may correct structural damage, but none of these replace the body's own repair intelligence. Without strengthening repair capacity, disease tends to recur or shift from one form to another.

Another simple example is maintaining personal finances. Occasional expenses are normal, but financial collapse occurs only when income, savings, and budgeting systems fail. A person does not go bankrupt because of one expense, but because the system that manages money is weak. Similarly, the body does not fail because of one injury or infection, but because the systems that manage repair, detoxification, and regeneration are overwhelmed or neglected. Strengthening these systems provides resilience against future stress.

The practical implication of this understanding is profound. Health care must shift from being crisis-oriented to maintenance-oriented. Daily habits such as adequate sleep, proper nutrition, regular movement, mental relaxation, and seasonal cleansing are not optional lifestyle choices; they are maintenance protocols for the human machine. When these are respected, the body tolerates stress, heals injuries, and adapts to change with remarkable efficiency.

In conclusion, healing is not a battle against disease but a process of restoring intelligent self-repair. Just as engineers prioritize maintenance to extend the life of machines, medicine must prioritize repair engineering to preserve human health. When repair capacity is protected and strengthened, damage remains manageable, aging slows, and disease becomes the exception rather than the rule.

Chapter 8

Predictive Maintenance & Disease Prevention Engineering

8.1 Introduction

In advanced engineering, the highest level of intelligence is not seen in how a system is repaired after failure, but in how effectively failure is prevented in the first place. Modern aircraft engines, power plants, and space systems operate under extreme conditions, yet they rarely fail suddenly because they are continuously monitored. Small changes in temperature, vibration, pressure, or efficiency are detected early, long before visible damage occurs. Engineers understand that breakdown is only the final event in a long chain of ignored warnings. Human biology follows the same principle. Disease does not appear suddenly on the day a report turns abnormal; it is the end result of months or years of unnoticed or neglected imbalance. Predictive health means recognizing that the body, like any advanced system, always warns before it breaks down.

Modern healthcare, however, often behaves like an emergency repair workshop rather than a preventive engineering unit. People usually seek medical attention only when pain becomes unbearable, when laboratory values cross abnormal limits, or when imaging shows visible structural damage. By this stage, the disease has already progressed deeply into the system. For example, a heart attack is often considered a sudden event, yet the arteries have been slowly accumulating damage for decades through inflammation, poor diet, stress, and metabolic imbalance. Similarly, diabetes is diagnosed when blood sugar crosses a threshold, even though insulin resistance and metabolic stress may have been present silently for many years. This reactive approach focuses on controlling damage rather than preventing it, much like repairing a collapsed bridge instead of strengthening it when small cracks first appear.

The human body, by design, is not a passive machine waiting to fail. It is an intelligent, self-monitoring system that constantly communicates its internal state. Early warning signals appear in simple, everyday forms such as persistent fatigue, loss of enthusiasm, irregular appetite, bloating, disturbed sleep, frequent mood changes, or reduced tolerance to stress. These signs are often dismissed as "normal," "due to age," or "part of a busy life," but in reality, they are the body's predictive alerts. For instance, repeated acidity and heaviness after meals is not just a digestive complaint; it is an early indication that metabolism is struggling. Ignoring such signals is similar to ignoring a warning light on a vehicle dashboard—movement may continue for some time, but internal damage quietly progresses.

Ayurveda recognized this predictive intelligence of the body thousands of years ago through the concept of Shatkriyakala, the six-stage progression of disease explained in the **Charaka Samhita**. This framework explains that disease begins at a subtle functional level, long before it becomes measurable or visible. In the early stages, imbalance exists only in physiological rhythm and energy flow, making it completely reversible with simple corrections. For example, irregular eating and late nights may initially cause mild tiredness and digestive discomfort. If these are corrected early, health is restored easily. If ignored, the same imbalance gradually advances toward hormonal disturbance, metabolic disease, and structural damage. Ayurveda emphasized that true medical intelligence lies in recognizing and correcting disease at these early stages, not waiting for full manifestation.

A simple example can be seen in joint health. Knee arthritis is often diagnosed when pain becomes severe and X-rays show cartilage loss.

However, years before this diagnosis, the person may have experienced morning stiffness, cracking sounds, heaviness, or reduced flexibility. These early signs indicate lubrication loss and tissue stress, not permanent damage. At this stage, proper diet, weight management, oil application, exercise correction, and rest can completely prevent progression. Once cartilage is destroyed, treatment becomes difficult and lifelong. Predictive maintenance focuses on acting during stiffness, not waiting for deformity, just as engineers lubricate moving parts before friction causes irreversible wear.

Another clear example is mental and emotional health. Anxiety disorders, depression, and burnout rarely appear suddenly. They develop gradually through chronic stress, poor sleep, irregular routines, and unresolved emotional strain. Early signs include irritability, poor concentration, disturbed sleep, and loss of motivation. When these are ignored, the nervous system slowly loses its ability to self-regulate, eventually leading to clinical disease. Ayurveda viewed these early mental disturbances as signals of imbalance that require lifestyle correction, nervous system calming, and rhythm restoration. Addressing them early prevents long-term psychiatric illness, proving again that predictive care is far more effective than crisis management.

In essence, predictive maintenance in human health is about shifting perspective—from treating disease as an unexpected enemy to understanding it as a predictable outcome of ignored signals. The body does not fail without warning; it communicates continuously through subtle changes long before breakdown occurs. Ayurveda provided a structured map to recognize these early stages and intervene intelligently, while modern medicine is only now beginning to acknowledge the value of early biomarkers and preventive strategies. When healthcare respects this predictive design, disease prevention becomes natural, economical, and sustainable, transforming medicine from damage control into true health engineering.

Predictive maintenance in human biology means understanding that the body, like any advanced machine, does not fail suddenly. In engineering, sensors constantly track small changes in temperature, vibration, pressure, or output efficiency. These minor deviations are early indicators that a component is under stress. If corrected early, failure is prevented. The human body functions on the same principle. Symptoms such as mild fatigue, frequent acidity, bloating, disturbed sleep, mood swings, or reduced stamina are not random discomforts; they are biological warning signals. They indicate that internal systems—digestion, metabolism, hormones, nerves, or immunity—are being overloaded or misused. Predictive health focuses on identifying and correcting these signals early, before they progress into irreversible disease.

In everyday life, people often ignore these early signals because they do not appear serious. A person may feel tired every morning, need excessive caffeine, experience irregular bowel habits, or notice gradual weight gain, yet continue normal routines, assuming these are "normal" effects of age or stress. From a predictive maintenance perspective, this is similar to ignoring a machine that is consuming slightly more fuel or producing slightly less output. The machine still runs, but efficiency is declining. In the body, declining efficiency appears as low energy, poor recovery, or reduced mental clarity. If lifestyle and habits are corrected at this stage, full efficiency can be restored. If ignored, the body compensates temporarily, but hidden damage continues to accumulate.

A simple layman's example is digestion. Occasional indigestion is common, but frequent acidity, heaviness after meals, or gas indicates that digestive capacity is weakening. This is not yet a disease, but it is an early deviation from normal function. If a person continues overeating, eating late at night, or consuming incompatible foods, the digestive system becomes chronically stressed. Over time, this can lead to metabolic disorders such as obesity, diabetes, or fatty liver. Predictive maintenance would involve correcting meal timing, portion size, and food quality at the stage of acidity itself, preventing the later development of serious disease.

Another common example is physical endurance. Reduced exercise tolerance—such as breathlessness while climbing stairs or early fatigue during routine activity—is often dismissed as lack of fitness. In predictive terms, this indicates declining cardiovascular or metabolic efficiency. Just as engineers investigate reduced performance output before machinery fails, the body requires early intervention through activity correction, stress reduction, and nutrition optimization. Waiting until chest pain or abnormal reports appear is equivalent to waiting for an engine to seize before servicing it. Early correction preserves long-term performance.

Mental and emotional symptoms are also powerful predictive indicators. Unexplained anxiety, irritability, poor sleep, or lack of motivation signal nervous system overload. These are often treated symptomatically with stimulants or sedatives, which suppress the warning without correcting the cause. Predictive maintenance instead asks why the nervous system is overstressed—irregular routine, excessive screen exposure, chronic stress, or lack of rest. Addressing these root factors early prevents progression into anxiety disorders, depression, or burnout, which are far more difficult to reverse.

In summary, predictive maintenance in human biology means respecting symptoms as intelligent messages, not inconveniences to be silenced. Disease does not begin with diagnosis; it begins when early warnings are ignored repeatedly. Mild fatigue today may become hormonal imbalance tomorrow and chronic disease later. Predictive health requires awareness, timely correction, and lifestyle discipline, just as engineering systems require monitoring, calibration, and scheduled servicing. Listening to the body early preserves health naturally, while suppression of signals only delays and deepens future breakdown.

8.2 Ayurvedic Framework: Shatkriyakala (Six Stages of Disease)

Ayurveda explains that every disease progresses through six predictable stages, beginning with subtle imbalance and ending in full structural damage. In the early stages, imbalance exists only at a functional or energetic level, with no abnormal test reports. For instance, repeated late-night meals may first cause heaviness and sluggish digestion. If ignored, this progresses to acidity, weight gain, insulin resistance, and finally diabetes or heart disease. Modern medicine usually intervenes at the fifth or sixth stage, when complications appear and lifelong medication becomes necessary. Ayurveda intervenes optimally in the first three stages, where simple lifestyle correction, diet regulation, and detoxification can completely reverse the process. This is the essence of predictive maintenance applied to human health.

8.3 Modern Predictive Medicine: A Parallel Evolution

Modern predictive medicine represents a significant shift from symptom-based treatment toward early risk detection and prevention, closely aligning with principles long established in Ayurveda. Instead of waiting for a disease to declare itself through pain or organ damage, modern science now studies subtle biochemical changes that appear years earlier. For example, HbA1c can identify prediabetes long before a person develops classic symptoms such as excessive thirst or frequent urination. At this stage, blood sugar may appear "almost normal," yet the body is already struggling with insulin efficiency. This is similar to detecting reduced fuel efficiency in an engine before it completely breaks down. Early identification allows simple lifestyle correction to reverse the process rather than lifelong medication after diabetes sets in.

Low-grade inflammation is another area where modern predictive medicine mirrors Ayurvedic insight. Markers such as hs-CRP detect silent inflammation that does not cause pain but slowly damages blood vessels and tissues. A person with elevated hs-CRP may feel outwardly healthy, yet internally, the groundwork for heart disease or metabolic disorder is being laid. Ayurveda described this stage as a hidden imbalance, where disease exists at a subtle level without obvious symptoms. If anti-inflammatory lifestyle measures such as proper diet, stress reduction, sleep correction, and detoxification are applied early, disease progression can be stopped. Ignoring this stage is like allowing corrosion to continue inside a pipe simply because there is no visible leak yet.

Imaging technology has further strengthened the predictive approach. Tests such as coronary calcium scoring can reveal plaque formation in arteries years before a heart attack occurs, while bone mineral density scans detect bone weakening before fractures happen. In daily life, this can be compared to detecting cracks inside a building's foundation before walls collapse. A person with early bone density loss may not feel pain, but predictive detection allows timely correction through nutrition, exercise, and hormonal balance. Waiting until a fracture occurs means structural damage has already taken place, requiring prolonged treatment and recovery.

Genetic and epigenetic profiling has added another powerful layer to predictive medicine. Certain individuals carry genetic tendencies that increase their vulnerability to specific diseases, but genes alone do not determine destiny. Lifestyle choices such as diet, physical activity, stress management, and sleep can switch genes on or off through epigenetic mechanisms. This explains why two people following similar habits may experience very different health outcomes. Ayurveda described this individual variability through the concept of Prakriti, or constitutional type, which determines how a person responds to food, climate, stress, and activity. Kha-vaigunya further explains why certain organs become weak points where disease manifests first.

A simple example is weight gain. Two people may consume similar diets, yet one gains weight rapidly while the other remains lean. Modern science may explain this through insulin sensitivity, genetic metabolism, or gut microbiome differences. Ayurveda explains it through constitutional differences and organ vulnerability. Predictive medicine does not apply the same solution to both individuals; instead, it personalizes intervention. One person may need carbohydrate regulation and stress reduction, while another may require digestive strengthening and routine stabilization. This personalized approach prevents disease instead of reacting to it later.

In essence, modern predictive medicine and Ayurveda are moving toward the same goal through different languages. Both recognize that disease begins long before diagnosis and that early, individualized intervention is the most effective form of healthcare. Biomarkers, imaging, and genetic tools provide modern confirmation of ancient wisdom that health must be monitored continuously, not episodically. When prediction replaces reaction and personalization replaces uniform treatment, medicine evolves from crisis management into true preventive engineering of health.

8.4 Clinical Example: Predictive Failure vs Preventive Intervention

A reactive clinical approach often creates the illusion that serious diseases occur suddenly, when in reality they represent the final stage of a long, predictable process. In the example of a 45-year-old man presenting with chest pain and being diagnosed with a myocardial infarction, the event appears abrupt only because earlier signals were ignored. For several years prior, the body had already been communicating distress through chronic fatigue, gradual weight gain, disturbed sleep, reduced enthusiasm for physical activity, and increasing dependence on stimulants such as tea or coffee. These signs indicated rising stress load, declining metabolic efficiency, and increasing inflammatory burden. From a biological engineering perspective, the heart attack was not the beginning of the disease but the endpoint of prolonged neglect.

From a layman's viewpoint, this situation is similar to a vehicle that suddenly breaks down on the highway. The owner may describe the failure as unexpected, yet the vehicle may have been consuming more fuel, making unusual noises, overheating slightly, and showing warning lights for months. Because it continued to function, servicing was postponed. In the human body, borderline cholesterol levels, mild blood pressure elevation, and poor sleep are equivalent to these early warning signs. They do not stop daily activity, so they are often ignored. However, internally, arteries are slowly accumulating inflammation and plaque, setting the stage for a major cardiac event.

A predictive engineering approach would view the same individual very differently. Instead of waiting for chest pain, assessment would occur when the early imbalance first appeared. Persistent fatigue would prompt evaluation of sleep quality, stress levels, and nervous system overload. Gradual weight gain would be recognized as a metabolic warning, not merely a cosmetic issue. Borderline cholesterol would be interpreted as an early vascular stress signal rather than something to be "watched" passively. This approach acknowledges that the body always signals distress early, and that intervention at this stage is both simpler and more effective.

Preventive intervention in such a case does not require extreme measures or lifelong medication. Simple dietary correction to reduce inflammatory and incompatible foods, structured exercise tailored to the individual's capacity, and stress unloading through routine regulation can dramatically reduce disease risk. Panchakarma detoxification, when applied at the stage of early imbalance, helps clear metabolic waste and restore physiological rhythm. At this point, arteries are still flexible, inflammation is reversible, and the heart muscle is not yet damaged. Just as timely servicing can extend the life of a machine for decades, early biological maintenance can preserve cardiovascular health long term.

Another important aspect of this example is the role of stress. Work-related pressure, irregular schedules, and mental strain often precede heart disease by many years. Stress does not damage the heart overnight; it gradually disrupts hormonal balance, sleep rhythm, digestion, and immune regulation. Over time, this creates a biochemical environment that accelerates vascular damage. In a reactive model, stress is addressed only after disease occurs. In a predictive model, stress is treated as a primary load factor, similar to excessive weight on a bridge. Reducing load early prevents structural failure later.

The contrast between predictive failure and preventive intervention highlights a critical truth: outcomes differ not because of chance, but because of timing. When intervention occurs late, treatment becomes complex, costly, and lifelong. When intervention occurs early, correction is simple, natural, and restorative. The heart attack in this example was not unavoidable; it was the result of missed opportunities for early maintenance. Predictive healthcare trains both physicians and individuals to recognize these opportunities and act before damage becomes permanent.

In summary, this clinical example demonstrates that disease progression follows a logical and predictable pathway. The body does not betray us suddenly; it warns repeatedly and patiently. Predictive engineering listens to these warnings and responds early, while reactive medicine responds only after collapse. The difference between these two approaches determines whether health is preserved or disease becomes a lifelong burden.

8.5 Preventive Engineering Tools in Ayurveda

Engineering tools in Ayurveda are designed on the same logic that keeps complex machines functioning smoothly over long periods of time. Just as machines require regular care even when they appear to be working well, the human body requires systematic maintenance to prevent future breakdown. Ayurveda does not wait for disease to appear; instead, it prescribes daily, seasonal, and individualized routines that continuously correct minor imbalances before they accumulate into illness. These routines are not rituals but practical biological maintenance protocols aimed at preserving efficiency, resilience, and longevity.

Dinacharya, or daily routine, functions like daily lubrication and calibration of a machine. In engineering, even the most advanced equipment requires daily checks to prevent friction, overheating, or misalignment. Similarly, the human body needs regular sleep, timely meals, proper elimination, and nervous system calming to function optimally. Going to bed late, skipping meals, or suppressing natural urges may not cause immediate disease, but they slowly disrupt biological rhythms. For example, a person who sleeps irregularly may initially experience only fatigue and irritability, but over time, this can lead to hormonal imbalance, poor digestion, and weakened immunity. Daily oil application, or Abhyanga, acts like lubrication for joints, nerves, and tissues, reducing wear and tear caused by stress and aging.

Ritucharya, or seasonal adaptation, is comparable to seasonal servicing of machines. Engineers change lubricants, adjust load, or modify operating conditions according to the climate to prevent predictable damage. The human body is equally sensitive to seasonal changes. Cold seasons increase stiffness, dryness, and respiratory issues, while hot seasons increase dehydration, acidity, and inflammation. Ayurveda advises changing diet, activity, and daily habits with each season to maintain balance. For instance, consuming warming, nourishing foods in winter prevents joint pain and immunity loss, while lighter, cooling foods in summer prevent heat-related digestive and skin disorders. Ignoring seasonal adaptation is like running the same engine settings in extreme heat and extreme cold—failure becomes only a matter of time.

Prakriti-based customization represents one of Ayurveda's most advanced preventive engineering tools. In mechanical systems, no two machines are operated exactly the same way; each has its own load capacity, fuel requirement, and tolerance limits. Ayurveda applies the same principle to human beings through the concept of individual constitution. A Kapha-dominant person naturally has stability and endurance but is prone to weight gain and sluggish metabolism if overnourished. Such individuals benefit from lighter meals, regular physical activity, and stimulation. In contrast, a Vata-dominant person is naturally active and creative but prone to dryness, anxiety, and degeneration. They require warmth, regular routines, nourishing food, and adequate rest. Applying the same diet or exercise plan to both individuals would be inefficient and potentially harmful.

Preventive tools in Ayurveda also emphasize timing and moderation rather than extremes. Machines fail faster when pushed continuously at maximum capacity without rest. Similarly, humans develop disease when they ignore the need for recovery. Regular meal timing supports digestive efficiency, just as regular fuel supply maintains engine stability. Proper elimination prevents toxin accumulation, similar to waste removal systems in machinery. When these daily functions are respected, the body maintains internal cleanliness and balance without requiring aggressive intervention later.

A simple example is office work. Two individuals may perform the same job, but one develops back pain, acidity, and stress-related illness while the other remains healthy. The difference often lies in daily routine, seasonal adaptation, and individual suitability. One may skip meals, sit for long hours, and sleep late, while the other maintains regular meals, stretches, and adequate rest. Ayurveda recognizes that preventive care must fit the individual and environment, not just the disease. This approach prevents problems before they appear, rather than treating them after they become severe.

In summary, preventive engineering tools in Ayurveda create a continuous maintenance system for the human body. Dinacharya preserves daily efficiency, Ritucharya protects against seasonal stress, and Prakriti-based customization ensures individual compatibility. Together, they form a predictive healthcare model that prevents disease by respecting biological design limits. Just as machines last longer with intelligent servicing, human health is preserved when these preventive principles are applied consistently and early.

8.6 Predictive Signals Commonly Ignored

Predictive signals commonly ignored are the earliest messages through which the body communicates internal imbalance. These signals are often mild, painless, and nonspecific, which is why they are easily dismissed as normal effects of aging, workload, or modern lifestyle. Persistent bloating, irregular appetite, acidity, disturbed sleep, frequent colds, mood fluctuations, morning stiffness, or reduced concentration are not random complaints. They reflect early dysfunction in digestion, immunity, hormonal rhythm, or nervous system regulation. In engineering terms, these are minor deviations in performance parameters, not failures. Treating them as insignificant allows the imbalance to deepen silently until it crosses the threshold of disease.

A common example is frequent digestive discomfort. Many people experience daily bloating, gas, or heaviness after meals and consider it normal. However, this indicates declining digestive efficiency and improper metabolic processing. Initially, this imbalance affects only comfort, but over time, it leads to toxin accumulation, weight gain, insulin resistance, and inflammatory disorders. If corrected early through proper meal timing, food selection, and portion control, digestion normalizes easily. Ignoring it is similar to allowing waste to accumulate in a machine's filtration system—performance gradually declines until a major breakdown occurs.

Frequent infections such as repeated colds, sore throats, or slow wound healing are another commonly ignored predictive signal. These are often attributed to weather changes or weak immunity without deeper evaluation. In reality, they indicate early immune exhaustion caused by poor sleep, chronic stress, nutritional deficiency, or improper daily routine. At this stage, immunity can be restored with rest, nourishment, and routine correction. If ignored, an immune imbalance may progress into chronic allergies, autoimmune disorders, or recurrent infections requiring long-term medication. Early correction prevents this downward spiral.

Mental and emotional changes are equally important predictive indicators. Irritability, anxiety, lack of motivation, forgetfulness, or disturbed sleep are often normalized as stress-related issues. However, these signs reflect early overload of the nervous system and hormonal imbalance. When addressed early through routine stabilization, stress reduction, and adequate rest, nervous balance is restored naturally. When ignored, the same imbalance progresses into anxiety disorders, depression, hypertension, or metabolic disease. Suppressing these signals with stimulants or sedatives is equivalent to silencing an alarm without fixing the underlying problem.

Musculoskeletal signals such as stiffness on waking, mild joint discomfort, or cracking sounds are frequently dismissed as age-related. These are early indicators of reduced lubrication, poor circulation, or tissue degeneration. At this stage, simple measures like regular movement, oil application, hydration, and seasonal care can fully reverse the process. If ignored, stiffness progresses into chronic pain, arthritis, and restricted mobility. From a preventive engineering perspective, lubrication and alignment are done before friction causes permanent damage, not after parts wear out.

Ayurveda emphasized the importance of recognizing these early warning signs long before modern medicine adopted preventive thinking. Classical texts such as the **Charaka Samhita** describe that disease becomes strong only when early signals are neglected and harmful habits are repeatedly continued. The body does not suddenly fail; it gradually loses balance through ignored messages. Predictive healthcare trains individuals to respect these messages as guidance rather than inconvenience.

In summary, predictive signals are not symptoms to be suppressed but information to be understood. They represent a valuable opportunity for correction at a stage where disease is still reversible. Ignoring them is like driving a vehicle with warning lights taped over the dashboard—movement continues temporarily, but damage accumulates silently. Recognizing and correcting these signals early preserves health, reduces suffering, and prevents the need for aggressive treatment later.

8.7 Disease as a Failure of Maintenance, Not Fate

Ayurveda clearly states that disease is not an unavoidable destiny written into the body, nor is it merely the result of faulty genes. Instead, disease is viewed as a gradual failure of maintenance. According to classical Ayurvedic understanding, the human body is inherently intelligent, adaptive, and self-regulating. As explained in the **Sushruta Samhita**, disease does not suddenly become powerful on its own; it gains strength only when it is repeatedly nourished by improper lifestyle, faulty diet, chronic stress, and neglect of early warning signs. This perspective shifts responsibility away from fear and fate and places it on daily choices and maintenance practices.

From a layman's point of view, this concept can be easily understood through everyday examples. A house does not collapse simply because it is old; it collapses because small cracks were ignored, water seepage was not repaired, and regular maintenance was neglected. Similarly, the body does not fall ill because it is weak, but because repeated signals of imbalance were overlooked. Occasional fatigue, disturbed sleep, mild pain, or digestive discomfort are not diseases, but they are early maintenance alerts. When these alerts are ignored and unhealthy habits continue, the imbalance deepens and eventually manifests as a diagnosable disease.

Modern thinking often labels diseases as "genetic" or "age-related," which can create helplessness in patients. While genetics may create vulnerability, they do not operate in isolation. Two individuals may carry similar genetic tendencies, yet only one develops disease because of differences in lifestyle, stress handling, diet, and routine. Ayurveda explained this long ago by emphasizing that causes must repeatedly act on a weak point for disease to develop. If maintenance is performed regularly, even a vulnerable system can function efficiently for a long time. This is why many people with genetic risk never develop disease, while others with no known genetic risk do.

Symptom suppression without correcting root causes is one of the most common reasons disease becomes chronic. Painkillers may reduce pain, antacids may suppress acidity, and stimulants may mask fatigue, but none of these correct the underlying imbalance. This is comparable to silencing a fire alarm without extinguishing the fire. The alarm stops making noise, giving a false sense of safety, while damage continues silently. Ayurveda emphasizes that symptoms are not enemies; they are messengers indicating where maintenance is required. Ignoring the message only allows the problem to grow deeper and more complex.

Another important aspect is the concept of preventive windows. Disease does not move from health to severe illness in one step. There are multiple stages where reversal is easy and natural. Missing these windows is what converts simple imbalance into serious pathology. For example, early metabolic imbalance can be corrected with diet and routine alone, but once diabetes develops, lifelong management becomes necessary. The body was not weak in the beginning; it simply was not maintained at the right time. Respecting these preventive windows is the core of disease prevention engineering.

When maintenance is respected, the body's innate intelligence works continuously to restore balance. Proper sleep resets the nervous system, correct diet restores metabolism, regular movement maintains circulation, and timely elimination removes waste. Under these conditions, resilience remains high and disease struggles to take root. Ayurveda's message is empowering: health is not a matter of luck, and disease is not fate. Most illnesses are the result of delayed maintenance, not defective design.

In summary, Ayurveda reframes disease as a failure of maintenance rather than an unavoidable outcome. The body is designed to remain healthy when its signals are respected and its needs are met on time. Disease strengthens only when early warnings are ignored and unhealthy patterns are repeated. By understanding this principle, healthcare shifts from fear-based treatment to responsibility-based prevention, allowing individuals to preserve health through intelligent, continuous maintenance of the human system.

An integrative predictive maintenance model represents a practical fusion of ancient Ayurvedic insight with modern medical technology. Instead of choosing between traditional wisdom and contemporary diagnostics, this model uses the strengths of both systems to protect health at its earliest stages. Ayurveda provides the conceptual framework to understand individuality, daily rhythm, and early imbalance, while modern medicine offers objective tools such as laboratory markers and imaging to confirm subtle changes. Together, they create a comprehensive system that detects risk early and guides timely correction, rather than waiting for disease to become clinically obvious.

The first step in this model is understanding the individual, not just the disease. Ayurveda begins with an assessment of constitution, lifestyle habits, mental stress, sleep patterns, digestion, and daily routine. This helps explain why the same environment or diet affects people differently. For example, two individuals working the same job may respond very differently to stress—one develops acidity and anxiety, while another gains weight and becomes sluggish. Modern diagnostics alone may not explain this difference, but constitutional assessment provides clarity. When this personalized understanding is combined with baseline investigations, healthcare becomes predictive rather than generic.

The second step involves identifying early imbalance using both subjective symptoms and objective markers. Ayurveda places importance on early functional changes such as loss of appetite rhythm, fatigue, disturbed sleep, or mood changes. Modern medicine complements this with biomarkers like blood sugar trends, inflammatory markers, lipid ratios, or early imaging changes. For instance, a person with normal reports but persistent tiredness and poor sleep is already showing an imbalance. Recognizing this stage allows intervention before reports turn abnormal. This dual observation ensures that neither symptoms nor numbers are ignored.

Timely correction is the core strength of the integrative predictive model. At early stages, correction is simple and restorative rather than aggressive. Dietary adjustment restores metabolic balance, routine regulation stabilizes biological clocks, stress management unloads the nervous system, and personalized exercise improves circulation and resilience. Detoxification, when applied appropriately, helps remove accumulated metabolic waste that blocks normal physiology. These interventions are not treatments for disease but maintenance tools to restore balance, similar to cleaning and recalibrating a system before damage occurs.

A simple example is seen in lifestyle-related metabolic disorders. A person with early weight gain, borderline blood sugar, and fatigue does not yet have diabetes. In a crisis-based model, no action may be taken until sugar levels rise further. In an integrative predictive model, this stage is recognized as a reversible imbalance. With diet correction, daily routine stabilization, stress reduction, and detox support, metabolism can normalize. This prevents progression to diabetes and avoids lifelong dependency on medication. The same principle applies to joint degeneration, digestive disorders, and stress-related illnesses.

This approach shifts healthcare away from crisis management toward continuous optimization. Instead of asking, "What disease do you have?" the focus becomes, "How well is your system functioning today?" Regular assessment and small corrections maintain efficiency and resilience. This philosophy is clearly described in **Ashtanga Hridaya**, which emphasizes daily and seasonal care, individualized living, and early correction as the foundation of health. The goal is not merely the absence of disease, but sustained balance and functional excellence.

In summary, the integrative predictive maintenance model treats the human body as a dynamic, intelligent system that requires continuous care. By combining Ayurvedic principles of individuality and early imbalance with modern diagnostic precision, healthcare becomes proactive, personalized, and preventive. Disease prevention becomes a natural outcome of intelligent maintenance rather than a constant battle against breakdown. This model represents the future of healthcare—one that preserves health by acting early, gently, and intelligently.

8.8 Key Takeaway: Redefining Healthcare

Redefining healthcare begins with changing the goal of medicine itself. In conventional systems, success is often measured by how effectively emergencies are managed, how accurately diseases are labeled, or how long a patient can be maintained on medication. While these interventions are important and sometimes lifesaving, they represent late-stage responses. True healthcare begins much earlier, when the body is still functional and imbalance is mild and reversible. Predictive healthcare focuses on identifying risk before damage occurs, much like engineers strengthen a structure before cracks widen. This approach preserves health rather than merely controlling disease.

A major limitation of disease-centered healthcare is lifelong dependency on drugs. When imbalance is detected late, medicines become necessary to compensate for lost function. For example, once diabetes is fully established, blood sugar often requires lifelong control. However, years before diagnosis, the body shows warning signs such as fatigue after meals, weight gain, poor sleep, or rising sugar trends. Addressing these early through diet, routine, and stress correction can prevent diabetes altogether. In this sense, lifelong medication often reflects missed preventive opportunities rather than an unavoidable destiny.

Personalization is another defining feature of true healthcare. Human beings differ in digestion, metabolism, stress tolerance, and recovery capacity. Treating everyone with the same diet advice, exercise plan, or medication dose ignores these differences and leads to poor outcomes. Predictive and preventive care adapts recommendations to the individual. For instance, a physically strong person may thrive on intense exercise, while another may develop exhaustion and injury from the same routine. Personalized care respects biological limits, just as engineers respect load limits for different machines. This reduces harm and enhances long-term effectiveness.

The role of the physician must therefore evolve. A repair technician intervenes only after a breakdown, replacing parts or suppressing malfunctions. A human body engineer, on the other hand, understands how the system works, where it is vulnerable, and how it should be maintained daily. Such a physician educates individuals about early warning signs, maintenance routines, and safe operating limits. This transforms patients from passive recipients of treatment into active partners in health preservation.

A simple understanding is household maintenance. A family that regularly checks wiring, plumbing, and roofing rarely faces disasters. Another family that ignores small leaks and cracks eventually faces flooding or collapse. Emergency repair may save the house temporarily, but prevention would have avoided the crisis altogether. Similarly, healthcare that waits for heart attacks, strokes, or organ failure is far costlier—physically, emotionally, and financially—than healthcare that prevents these outcomes through early action.

Ultimately, the most advanced medical system is not defined by dramatic rescues at the final stage of illness, but by the quiet absence of disease over a lifetime. Saving life at the last moment is noble, but preventing disease from ever taking root is far superior. When healthcare prioritizes prediction, prevention, and personalization, medicine fulfills its highest purpose—preserving vitality, function, and quality of life rather than merely delaying decline.

Chapter 9

The Human Body Is Not a Dumping Ground

Unhealthy Foods, Biological Consequences & Preventive Engineering

9.1 Introduction – Why the Body Was Never Designed to Handle Garbage

In engineering science, every machine is designed with a clearly defined input–output relationship. A high-performance system such as a jet engine, power turbine, or precision manufacturing robot is not built to tolerate random materials, contaminated fuel, or repeated misuse. Even if the machine is serviced regularly, wrong inputs slowly damage internal components, clog channels, reduce efficiency, and ultimately cause failure. Importantly, such failure does not occur suddenly; it develops silently over time until one day the system collapses. The same foundational engineering logic applies to the human body. The body is not a waste-processing plant meant to tolerate unlimited chemical exposure, artificial additives, or poorly designed food substitutes. It is a highly sensitive, precision-engineered biological system that functions optimally only when the quality, compatibility, quantity, and timing of its inputs are respected.

The human body operates with extraordinary intelligence, efficiency, and self-repair capacity, but this intelligence has biological limits. Just as a high-grade engine requires clean fuel, correct viscosity oil, and periodic calibration, the body requires food that it can recognize, digest, absorb, and integrate into living tissue. When repeatedly exposed to ultra-processed foods, chemical additives, synthetic sweeteners, and artificial fats, the body does not immediately collapse. Instead, it adapts temporarily by overworking digestive enzymes, hormonal systems, detoxification pathways, and immune defenses. From engineering view point using poor quality fuel in a vehicle; the car may run for years, but mileage drops, engine noise increases, parts wear out faster, and major repairs become inevitable. In the same way, people often feel "normal" while silent biological damage is accumulating underneath.

Modern medicine is currently witnessing an unprecedented rise in lifestyle and chronic diseases such as diabetes, obesity, heart disease, autoimmune disorders, infertility, depression, anxiety, and neurodegenerative conditions. This epidemic is not occurring because the human body has suddenly become weaker or less intelligent. Rather, it is occurring because modern food has become biologically abnormal. Human genetics have not changed significantly in the last few thousand years, but food processing methods, chemical exposure, and eating patterns have changed dramatically within just a few decades. The body is therefore forced to operate in an environment for which it was never designed. This mismatch between biological design and modern input is the root cause of many contemporary diseases.

Ayurveda articulated this principle thousands of years ago with remarkable clarity. In the **Charaka Samhita**, it is stated that *"Ahara Sambhavam Vastuh"*, meaning that the physical structure, strength, resilience, and disease tendencies of the body arise directly from the food consumed. This means that food is not just something that fills the stomach; it literally becomes blood, muscle, fat, bone, hormones, and even reproductive tissue. Over time, repeated dietary choices shape the body's metabolism, immunity, and aging pattern. What a person eats daily slowly but surely becomes their physical reality.

From a modern biological perspective, this ancient statement is now supported by scientific evidence. Food does not merely supply calories; it delivers biochemical signals that influence hormones, gut bacteria, immune responses, inflammation levels, and gene expression. Repeated exposure to refined sugar programs insulin resistance. Excess unhealthy fats reprogram cell membranes. Chemical additives interfere with neurotransmitters and hormones. A simple example is repeatedly watering a plant with polluted water. The plant may survive initially, but its leaves lose color, growth becomes stunted, and eventually the roots rot. Similarly, wrong food does not cause immediate illness but silently alters internal biology until disease appears.

In the modern world, humans routinely consume substances that the digestive system never evolved to handle. Ultra-processed foods, artificial colors, preservatives, trans fats, excessive sugar, and chemical residues are relatively new exposures in evolutionary terms. The digestive system is designed for fresh, seasonal, natural foods that spoil quickly, not for products that remain edible for months or years on shelves. When such unnatural foods are consumed repeatedly, digestion becomes overloaded, gut bacteria lose diversity, and metabolic waste begins to accumulate. Hormonal signals become confused, inflammation increases, and tissue repair mechanisms slow down. This explains why many people feel chronically tired, bloated, anxious, or unwell long before any laboratory diagnosis is made.

Psychologically, many modern foods are engineered to override natural satiety signals. Excess sugar, salt, and artificial flavor enhancers stimulate brain reward pathways, encouraging overconsumption. This creates eating patterns driven by craving rather than hunger. From an engineering analogy, this is like disabling a machine's warning sensors so it continues running despite overheating. The system keeps operating, but internal damage accelerates. In humans, this results in overeating, obesity, addiction-like behavior, and loss of intuitive eating intelligence.

This chapter is therefore essential to understanding disease prevention. It explains how inappropriate food acts as a slow poison rather than an immediate toxin, how Ayurveda interprets this process through concepts such as impaired digestion and metabolic waste, and how modern science explains the same process through inflammation, insulin resistance, microbiome disruption, and hormonal imbalance. Most importantly, it introduces the idea of preventive food engineering—choosing inputs intelligently so that disease can be avoided long before medicines or surgeries are required. Just as engineers protect machines by controlling input quality, human health can be protected by respecting the biological design principles of food and digestion.

9.2 Classification of Unhealthy Foods – Modern Science and Ayurvedic Perspective

9.2.1 Ultra-Processed Foods (UPFs)

Ultra-processed foods are industrially manufactured food products that are far removed from their original natural form. They include packaged snacks such as chips and wafers, instant noodles, processed meats like sausages and nuggets, sugary breakfast cereals, frozen ready-to-eat meals, soft drinks, and fast foods. These products are not created with the primary intention of nourishing the human body. Instead, they are engineered for long shelf life, intense taste stimulation, attractive appearance, and repeated consumption. To achieve this, manufacturers use refined carbohydrates, unhealthy fats, excessive salt, sugar, artificial flavors, colors, emulsifiers, and preservatives. During processing, most natural fibers, vitamins, minerals, and digestive enzymes are destroyed, leaving behind calories without biological intelligence.

From a modern scientific perspective, ultra-processed foods disturb the body at multiple levels simultaneously. Because they are rapidly digestible, they cause sudden spikes in blood glucose, forcing the pancreas to release large amounts of insulin. When this happens repeatedly, the body's cells become less responsive to insulin, leading to insulin resistance. At the same time, these foods lack fiber, which is essential for feeding healthy gut bacteria. As a result, the gut microbiome loses diversity, beneficial bacteria decrease, and harmful bacteria gain dominance. Since the gut microbiome plays a central role in immunity, metabolism, hormone regulation, and even brain function, its disruption creates widespread systemic imbalance.

Over time, regular consumption of ultra-processed foods leads to chronic low-grade inflammation throughout the body. This inflammation is not intense enough to cause immediate pain or fever, so it often goes unnoticed, but it slowly damages blood vessels, liver cells, pancreatic tissue, and joints. Weight gain occurs not only because of excess calories, but because metabolic signaling becomes faulty. Fatty liver disease develops when the liver is overloaded with refined sugars and unhealthy fats. Eventually, this silent damage manifests as obesity, type 2 diabetes, high blood pressure, heart disease, and even certain cancers. A simple example is continuously using low-quality fuel mixed with dirt in a car. The vehicle may run for years, but fuel efficiency drops, engine noise increases, parts wear out prematurely, and one day the engine fails unexpectedly.

Ultra-processed foods also interfere with natural appetite control. Because they are designed to be hyper-palatable, they override the body's satiety signals. A person may continue eating even after the body's nutritional needs are met, simply because taste receptors and brain reward pathways are overstimulated. This leads to habitual overeating without true hunger. In everyday terms, it is similar to watching television with the volume turned too high; over time, normal sound no longer feels sufficient, and louder input is constantly needed. In the same way, natural foods begin to feel "bland," pushing individuals toward increasingly processed options.

Ayurveda provides a clear and insightful explanation for the harmful effects of ultra-processed foods. These foods are classified as *Guru*, meaning heavy and difficult to digest, because they burden the digestive system without providing corresponding nourishment. They are also described as *Abhishyandi*, meaning substances that clog bodily channels. Such foods weaken *Agni*, the digestive and metabolic fire responsible for transforming food into usable energy and tissues. When *Agni* becomes weak or irregular, digestion remains incomplete, and *Ama*—toxic, sticky metabolic waste—is formed.

Once *Ama* is produced, it does not remain confined to the digestive tract. It circulates throughout the body and lodges in weak or overused tissues. In joints, it contributes to stiffness and pain; in blood vessels, it promotes blockage and poor circulation; in the liver, it causes fatty changes; and in metabolic tissues, it leads to disorders such as diabetes and obesity. Ayurveda explains that disease does not begin suddenly in an organ, but starts with impaired digestion and toxic accumulation long before symptoms appear. Thus, from both modern science and Ayurvedic understanding, ultra-processed foods act as slow poisons—substances that do not kill immediately, but quietly erode health over years of repeated consumption.

9.2.2 Refined Sugar and High-Glycemic Foods

Refined sugar and high glycemic foods represent one of the most significant nutritional threats in modern diets. These include white sugar, high fructose corn syrup, sweetened beverages, packaged fruit juices, bakery products made with refined flour, candies, desserts, and many commercially prepared sweets. These substances are rapidly absorbed into the bloodstream because they lack natural fiber and structural complexity. As a result, they cause sudden and excessive rises in blood glucose levels. To manage this surge, the pancreas is forced to release large amounts of insulin repeatedly. While this compensatory mechanism initially keeps blood sugar under control, constant overuse gradually exhausts insulin receptors, leading to insulin resistance and eventually type 2 diabetes.

From a layman's perspective, this process can be compared to continuously ringing a doorbell without pause. At first, the bell rings loudly and clearly, but with repeated overuse, the internal wiring overheats and fails. Similarly, insulin signaling becomes ineffective due to constant overstimulation. Over time, blood sugar remains elevated despite high insulin levels, creating a state where the body is both flooded with glucose and unable to use it efficiently. This metabolic confusion leads to fatigue, increased hunger, weight gain, and long-term organ damage.

Excess sugar intake also promotes oxidative stress, a condition where harmful free radicals damage cells, proteins, and DNA. Blood vessels are particularly vulnerable, leading to stiffening of arteries and increased risk of heart disease. The liver converts excess sugar, especially fructose, into fat, resulting in non-alcoholic fatty liver disease. Unlike dietary fat, sugar-derived fat accumulates silently in liver cells, gradually impairing liver function. A simple everyday example is pouring sugar syrup into a filter system designed for water; initially, it flows through, but over time, it clogs and damages the system.

Refined sugar also affects the brain in powerful ways. It stimulates dopamine release, the neurotransmitter associated with pleasure and reward. Repeated stimulation alters brain reward circuits, making individuals crave sugary foods even when they consciously understand the harm. This creates addiction-like behavior, where consumption is driven by craving rather than hunger. People often experience mood swings, irritability, and energy crashes after sugar intake, further reinforcing the cycle of repeated consumption. This explains why many individuals find it difficult to reduce sugar despite experiencing health problems.

Ayurveda provides a parallel explanation through the concept of excessive *Madhura Rasa* (sweet taste). While natural sweetness in moderation is nourishing, overconsumption leads to *Kapha* aggravation and excessive formation of *Meda* (fat tissue). This results in heaviness, lethargy, coldness, and fluid retention. Over time, metabolic pathways become clogged, leading to disorders classified under *Prameha*, which includes diabetes and related metabolic diseases. Ayurveda emphasizes that such disorders develop gradually, beginning with a subtle digestive imbalance long before clinical disease becomes evident.

Excessive intake of refined sugar also weakens *Agni*, the digestive and metabolic fire. Initially, sweetness may appear energizing, but over time, it dulls digestion, increases mucus production, and promotes toxic accumulation. This creates a vicious cycle in which poor digestion leads to increased craving for quick energy sources like sugar, further worsening metabolic imbalance. Thus, both modern medicine and Ayurveda converge on the same conclusion: refined sugar does not cause sudden illness, but silently programs the body toward metabolic disease, addiction, and premature aging through repeated and habitual consumption.

9.2.3 Trans Fats and Industrial Seed Oils

Trans fats and industrially processed seed oils represent one of the most harmful categories of dietary fats introduced in modern times. These fats are commonly found in vanaspati, margarine, commercial bakery shortenings, reused frying oils, packaged snacks, and fast foods. They are created through industrial processes such as hydrogenation and repeated high-temperature heating, which alter the natural structure of fats. As a result, these fats no longer resemble the natural oils that the human digestive and metabolic systems evolved to handle. Although they provide calories, they lack biological compatibility and act more like foreign substances within the body.

Modern scientific research shows that trans fats and damaged seed oils integrate directly into cell membranes. Healthy cell membranes are meant to be flexible and dynamic, allowing nutrients, oxygen, hormones, and waste products to move efficiently in and out of the cell. When rigid trans fats replace natural fats in these membranes, the membranes lose their flexibility and become stiff. This disrupts normal cellular communication, reduces nutrient exchange, and impairs cellular repair mechanisms. Over time, this cellular rigidity contributes to widespread inflammation, tissue degeneration, and premature aging.

From a layman's perspective, this process can be understood by imagining flexible rubber pipes being replaced with brittle plastic ones. Rubber pipes can bend and withstand pressure changes, whereas brittle plastic cracks easily under stress. Similarly, when blood vessels and cells lose flexibility due to unhealthy fats, circulation becomes impaired, pressure increases, and the risk of rupture or blockage rises. This explains why diets high in trans fats are strongly associated with coronary artery disease, strokes, and peripheral vascular disorders.

Industrial seed oils that are repeatedly heated, such as reused cooking oils in restaurants, undergo oxidation and form toxic byproducts. These oxidized fats generate free radicals that damage the lining of blood vessels and trigger immune responses. Chronic exposure keeps the body in a constant low-grade inflammatory state. This inflammation does not cause immediate symptoms but silently damages the heart, brain, joints, and kidneys. A simple everyday example is rust forming inside metal machinery; initially invisible, but eventually causing breakdown and failure.

Ayurveda explains the harmful effects of these fats through the concept of *Vikruta Sneha*. *Sneha* refers to nourishing fats that support lubrication, strength, and vitality when consumed in their natural form. However, when fats are chemically altered, overheated, or repeatedly reused, they lose their nourishing quality and become *Vikruta*, meaning distorted or unnatural. Such fats fail to nourish tissues properly and instead create blockage in bodily channels, a condition known as *Srotorodha*. When circulation through these channels is impaired, tissues are deprived of nourishment and waste products accumulate, accelerating degenerative changes.

According to Ayurvedic understanding, blocked channels disturb the flow of nutrients, oxygen, and life force, leading to weakness, stiffness, pain, and organ dysfunction. Over time, this contributes to diseases of aging such as heart disease, joint degeneration, neurological decline, and reduced vitality. Thus, both modern science and Ayurveda clearly indicate that trans fats and industrial seed oils do not simply add unhealthy calories; they fundamentally alter cellular structure and function. Their damage is slow, cumulative, and often irreversible, making them one of the most dangerous dietary inputs when consumed regularly.

9.2.4 Artificial Additives and Chemical Preservatives

Artificial additives and chemical preservatives are substances added to food not to nourish the body, but to improve taste, color, texture, and shelf life. Common examples include flavor enhancers such as monosodium glutamate (MSG), synthetic food colors like tartrazine, artificial sweeteners such as aspartame and saccharin, and preservatives like sodium benzoate and sulfites. These chemicals allow food to remain attractive and edible for long periods, often months or years, but they are substances the human digestive and metabolic systems were never designed to process regularly. While small amounts may not cause immediate harm, repeated and long-term exposure creates cumulative biological stress.

From a modern scientific standpoint, many of these additives interfere with fundamental cellular processes. Certain artificial additives are known to affect brain neurotransmitters, leading to neurotoxicity and altered nerve signaling. Others impair mitochondrial function, reducing the cell's ability to produce energy efficiently. Since mitochondria are the "power plants" of the cell, their dysfunction leads to fatigue, poor organ function, and accelerated aging. Some preservatives and sweeteners also interfere with hormonal signaling, confusing the endocrine system and disrupting appetite regulation, metabolism, and stress responses.

In children, the effects of artificial colors and flavor enhancers are particularly evident. Studies have shown that regular consumption of foods containing synthetic colors is associated with increased hyperactivity, restlessness, irritability, and difficulty concentrating. A simple example is giving a child a brightly colored sugary drink and observing sudden excitement followed by irritability and restlessness. This is not merely a behavioral issue but a biochemical reaction occurring in the brain. Because children's nervous systems are still developing, they are especially sensitive to chemical stimulation and toxicity.

In adults, long-term consumption of artificial additives manifests in more subtle but serious ways. Frequent headaches or migraines, unexplained mood swings, anxiety, sleep disturbances, digestive discomfort, and reduced immunity are commonly reported. Over time, chronic exposure may contribute to autoimmune disorders and increase long-term cancer risk by promoting oxidative stress and DNA damage. A relatable example is living in a polluted city; the effects are not immediately dramatic, but years of exposure gradually damage the lungs, heart, and overall vitality.

Ayurveda classifies such chemically modified substances under *Viruddha Ahara*, meaning incompatible or contradictory food. These are foods that may appear edible but are fundamentally unsuitable for the body's tissues and metabolic pathways. According to Ayurvedic principles, *Viruddha Ahara* disrupts digestion and creates toxic byproducts that circulate in the body. These substances particularly vitiate *Rakta* (blood tissue), leading to skin disorders, allergies, inflammatory conditions, and impaired circulation. When the blood is impure, nourishment to all tissues becomes faulty.

In addition to physical effects, Ayurveda emphasizes the mental and emotional consequences of incompatible foods. Artificial additives disturb mental balance, described as *Manasika Vikara*. This explains the increasing prevalence of anxiety, irritability, emotional instability, and depressive tendencies in populations consuming large amounts of chemically enhanced foods. Just as contaminated fuel affects not only engine parts but also electronic sensors and control systems, chemically adulterated food affects both the body and the mind. Thus, both modern science and Ayurveda clearly indicate that artificial additives and preservatives are not harmless conveniences, but slow-acting disruptors that undermine physical health, mental stability, and long-term well-being when consumed regularly.

9.2.5 Alcohol and Recreational Substances

Alcohol and other recreational substances occupy a unique position in modern society because they are widely accepted, socially normalized, and often even celebrated, despite being biologically toxic. Alcohol, in particular, is a substance that the human body recognizes as a poison. From the moment it enters the bloodstream, the body prioritizes its elimination over all other metabolic tasks. Modern medical science has clearly documented that alcohol damages nearly every organ system, with the liver and brain being the primary targets. Its hepatotoxic effects include fatty liver, hepatitis, fibrosis, and cirrhosis, while its neurotoxic effects lead to cognitive decline, memory impairment, mood disturbances, and neurodegeneration.

Even moderate but chronic alcohol consumption places continuous stress on the liver's detoxification pathways. The liver must convert alcohol into acetaldehyde, a highly toxic intermediate compound, before further breaking it down for elimination. Repeated exposure overwhelms this system, allowing toxic metabolites to accumulate and damage liver cells. Over time, the liver becomes less efficient at detoxifying other substances, including medications, environmental toxins, and metabolic waste. A simple example is a factory forced to handle hazardous waste nonstop; eventually, the machinery wears out, workers become inefficient, and the entire system begins to fail.

Alcohol also profoundly affects the brain and nervous system. It disrupts neurotransmitter balance, initially producing relaxation or euphoria, but later causing anxiety, irritability, sleep disturbances, and depression.

Chronic use shrinks brain volume, slows nerve conduction, and impairs decision-making and impulse control. This explains why long-term alcohol consumption is associated with poor judgment, emotional instability, and increased risk of accidents and violence. From an everyday perspective, this is similar to repeatedly short-circuiting an electrical control panel; it may function temporarily, but wiring damage accumulates until malfunction becomes inevitable.

The immune system is another major casualty of alcohol consumption. Alcohol suppresses immune cell function, reduces the body's ability to fight infections, and increases susceptibility to respiratory illnesses, tuberculosis, and slow wound healing. It also promotes chronic inflammation, which contributes to cardiovascular disease and increases the risk of multiple cancers, including liver, oral, esophageal, breast, and colorectal cancers. Importantly, these risks increase with cumulative exposure, meaning that even small daily amounts consumed over many years can produce serious long-term harm.

Ayurveda provides a deeply insightful explanation for these effects through the concept of *Madya*. While small quantities of alcohol may have specific medicinal or contextual uses, excessive or habitual consumption is considered highly destructive. Ayurveda states that alcohol leads to *Ojas Kshaya*, the depletion of *Ojas*, which is the vital essence responsible for immunity, strength, mental clarity, and longevity. When *Ojas* is diminished, the individual becomes prone to infections, fatigue, emotional instability, and premature aging. This concept closely parallels modern observations of immune suppression and systemic weakness in chronic alcohol users.

In addition, Ayurveda explains that alcohol vitiates *Rakta* (blood) and *Yakrit* (liver), leading to impaired circulation, poor tissue nourishment, and toxin accumulation. As liver function declines, digestion weakens, metabolism becomes erratic, and the body's natural repair mechanisms slow down. The analogy of using industrial solvent instead of engine oil is particularly apt here. While the engine may run briefly, internal components suffer severe damage due to lack of proper lubrication and corrosion. Similarly, alcohol may provide temporary relaxation or social comfort, but it gradually erodes the body's internal systems, leaving long-lasting and often irreversible damage. Thus, both modern medicine and Ayurveda agree that alcohol is not a harmless indulgence, but a slow-acting toxin that undermines physical health, mental balance, and biological resilience when consumed regularly.

9.2.6 Plastic-Packaged and Chemically Contaminated Foods

Plastic-packaged and chemically contaminated foods represent a hidden but highly significant source of chronic toxicity in modern life. Foods stored or heated in plastic containers, beverages kept in plastic bottles, vegetables grown with excessive pesticides, and water contaminated with heavy metals such as lead, mercury, and arsenic expose the human body to substances it was never designed to encounter on a daily basis. Chemicals like bisphenol-A (BPA), phthalates, pesticide residues, and heavy metals slowly enter the body through ingestion, even though their presence is often invisible, tasteless, and unnoticed.

From a modern scientific perspective, many of these chemicals act as endocrine disruptors, meaning they interfere with normal hormonal signaling. Hormones function at extremely small concentrations and control growth, metabolism, reproduction, mood, and development. When endocrine-disrupting chemicals mimic or block natural hormones, the body receives confused signals. This leads to menstrual irregularities, reduced sperm quality, infertility, thyroid dysfunction, early puberty in children, and metabolic disorders. A simple example is a faulty remote control sending wrong commands to a television; the screen flickers, changes channels randomly, or shuts down altogether.

Heavy metals such as lead and mercury cause additional damage by accumulating in tissues over time. These metals interfere with enzyme activity, damage nerve cells, impair kidney function, and disrupt brain development, especially in children. Unlike many toxins that are quickly eliminated, heavy metals persist in the body for years. Drinking contaminated water daily or consuming food grown in polluted soil is comparable to slowly filling a storage room with garbage—each day adds a small amount, but eventually the space becomes unusable. The danger lies not in immediate illness, but in long-term accumulation.

Heating food in plastic containers further worsens the problem. Heat increases the release of plastic-derived chemicals into food, especially oily or acidic items. Repeated exposure overwhelms the liver's detoxification capacity, leading to fatigue, headaches, hormonal imbalance, and increased cancer risk. Many people feel "unwell" without clear medical findings, unaware that their daily exposure to plastics and chemical residues is silently affecting their health. This explains the rise in unexplained chronic symptoms despite normal laboratory reports.

Ayurveda provides a remarkably accurate explanation for this phenomenon through the concept of *Dushi Visha*. *Dushi Visha* refers to low-grade, cumulative poisoning that does not cause immediate collapse like acute poisoning, but gradually weakens tissues, digestion, immunity, and mental clarity. Because symptoms develop slowly, individuals often fail to recognize the cause, allowing exposure to continue unchecked. Over time, this leads to chronic diseases such as skin disorders, hormonal imbalances, infertility, neurological issues, and cancers.

According to Ayurvedic understanding, *Dushi Visha* lodges in tissues, obstructs bodily channels, and weakens *Agni*, the digestive and metabolic fire. Once *Agni* is compromised, the body loses its ability to neutralize toxins effectively, allowing deeper tissue damage to occur. This mirrors modern observations of toxin bioaccumulation and impaired detox pathways. Thus, both modern science and Ayurveda warn that plastic-packaged and chemically contaminated foods pose a silent but serious threat. Their harm lies not in dramatic poisoning, but in slow, continuous exposure that gradually erodes health, vitality, and longevity without immediate warning signs.

9.3 Major Threats Arising from Unhealthy Food Consumption

Unhealthy food does not harm the body in isolation or target a single organ. Instead, it disrupts entire biological systems that are designed to work in coordination. The human body functions like an integrated network, where digestion, metabolism, immunity, hormones, the nervous system, and reproduction are deeply interconnected. When food quality is poor, artificial, or incompatible with human biology, the damage spreads across multiple systems simultaneously. This is why modern diseases rarely appear alone; obesity often coexists with diabetes, heart disease with depression, gut disorders with anxiety, and infertility with hormonal imbalance.

From a metabolic perspective, unhealthy food is a primary driver of obesity, diabetes, and lipid disorders. Ultra-processed foods, refined sugars, and unhealthy fats overload the body with excess calories while providing minimal nutrition. Metabolic signals that regulate hunger, satiety, and energy usage become confused. Fat storage increases while cellular energy utilization decreases, leading to weight gain even with normal or reduced food intake. A simple example is a factory receiving too much raw material but lacking skilled workers to process it; waste piles up, efficiency drops, and output quality declines. Similarly, the body accumulates fat while cells remain undernourished, resulting in fatigue, insulin resistance, and metabolic syndrome.

Immunologically, unhealthy food creates a constant state of low-grade inflammation. Excess sugar, trans fats, chemical additives, and gut-damaging foods stimulate immune cells continuously, even in the absence of infection. Over time, this chronic immune activation exhausts immune defenses and increases the risk of autoimmune diseases, allergies, and frequent infections. People may notice that they fall sick often, take longer to recover, or develop unexplained inflammatory conditions. This is comparable to an alarm system that is constantly triggered by false signals; eventually, it malfunctions and fails to respond appropriately to real threats.

Digestive disorders are among the earliest and most visible consequences of unhealthy eating. Poor-quality food disrupts digestive enzymes, weakens gut lining integrity, and alters the balance of gut bacteria. This leads to conditions such as irritable bowel syndrome, acid reflux, bloating, constipation, diarrhea, and non-alcoholic fatty liver disease. Gut dysbiosis—an imbalance between beneficial and harmful bacteria—

impairs nutrient absorption and toxin elimination. If we think on the principle of engineering a sewage treatment plant where helpful bacteria are destroyed; waste accumulates, foul gases form, and the entire system becomes inefficient. Since the gut is central to immunity and mental health, digestive dysfunction acts as a gateway to broader disease.

Neurologically and psychologically, unhealthy food has profound effects on brain function and emotional health. The brain depends on stable blood sugar, healthy fats, micronutrients, and a balanced gut microbiome. Diets high in refined sugar and artificial additives cause blood sugar fluctuations, neurotransmitter imbalance, and chronic inflammation in the brain. This contributes to depression, anxiety, irritability, poor concentration, memory decline, and addiction-like eating behavior. Many individuals experience mood swings, brain fog, or emotional instability without realizing that their diet is a major contributing factor. This is similar to running sensitive electronic equipment on an unstable power supply—performance becomes erratic, and failures increase.

Reproductive health is also highly sensitive to dietary quality. Unhealthy food disrupts hormonal balance, affects insulin signaling, and increases inflammatory load, leading to conditions such as polycystic ovarian syndrome, infertility, reduced sperm quality, menstrual irregularities, and early reproductive aging. In women, excess insulin and inflammation directly affect ovulation, while in men, toxin accumulation and oxidative stress impair sperm health. Beyond immediate fertility issues, unhealthy food can cause epigenetic changes—chemical modifications in DNA expression that do not alter genes themselves but influence how genes function. These changes can be passed to future generations, increasing their risk of obesity, diabetes, and metabolic disorders.

Overall, the major threat of unhealthy food lies in its silent, cumulative, and system-wide impact. Damage does not appear overnight or in a single organ; it unfolds gradually across metabolism, immunity, digestion, brain function, and reproduction. By the time a disease is diagnosed, multiple systems are often already compromised. This systemic nature of damage explains why treating one organ alone rarely restores health fully. True prevention and recovery require correcting the quality of food input so that all interconnected systems can regain balance and function as originally designed.

9.4 Ayurvedic Pathophysiology – How Wrong Food Creates Disease

According to classical Ayurvedic understanding described in **Charaka Samhita**, particularly in *Sutrasthana 28*, disease does not begin suddenly in an organ, nor does it arise randomly. Disease is the final visible stage of a long, silent internal process that starts with improper food and faulty digestion. Ayurveda explains this progression in a logical, stepwise manner that closely resembles modern concepts of subclinical disease, metabolic dysfunction, and chronic inflammation. This model emphasizes that wrong food harms the body first at the functional level, long before structural damage becomes detectable.

The first and most critical step in disease formation is *Agni Dushti*, or impairment of digestive and metabolic fire. *Agni* is not limited to stomach digestion alone; it represents the body's entire capacity to digest, transform, and assimilate food at every level—from the gut to individual cells. When food is heavy, artificial, incompatible, excessive, or consumed at improper times, *Agni* becomes weak, irregular, or erratic. A simple example is a cooking stove with a low or unstable flame. Even good ingredients will not cook properly if the flame is insufficient or fluctuating. Similarly, even nutritious food fails to nourish when digestion is impaired.

Once *Agni* is weakened, digestion becomes incomplete, leading to the formation of *Ama*. *Ama* is described as sticky, toxic, undigested metabolic waste that results from improper digestion. It is not immediately expelled from the body; instead, it accumulates silently. In modern terms, *Ama* can be compared to partially burned fuel residue or sludge that forms when combustion is inefficient. A layman's analogy is smoke and soot forming in a chimney when firewood is damp—initially unnoticed, but gradually clogging the passage and reducing efficiency.

After formation, *Ama* does not remain confined to the digestive tract. It enters circulation and begins to obstruct *Srotas*, the microscopic and macroscopic channels responsible for transporting nutrients, oxygen, hormones, and waste products throughout the body. This obstruction, known as *Srotorodha*, prevents proper nourishment of tissues and impairs waste removal. In everyday terms, this is like debris accumulating inside water pipes. At first, water flow slows slightly, but over time, pressure builds, leakage occurs, and supply to distant areas becomes inadequate.

As *Srotas* become blocked, individual tissues (*Dhatus*) begin to suffer. Each tissue has its own metabolic intelligence and nourishment requirements. When toxic residue interferes with this process, tissues become either deficient or excessively accumulated. Fat tissue may increase abnormally, muscles may weaken, blood quality may deteriorate, or bone strength may reduce. For example is soil contaminated with pollutants; some plants grow excessively as weeds, while useful crops fail to thrive. Tissue imbalance is therefore the foundation of visible disease.

Over time, the continued presence of *Ama* and tissue dysfunction leads to *Dosha* aggravation. *Vata*, *Pitta*, and *Kapha* lose their natural balance and begin to act pathologically. For example, blocked channels may provoke *Vata*, leading to pain and degeneration; toxic heat may aggravate *Pitta*, causing inflammation and ulcers; excessive heaviness may increase *Kapha*, resulting in obesity and lethargy. This stage corresponds to early functional disorders in modern medicine, where symptoms appear but structural damage may still be reversible.

If wrong food intake continues unchecked, the disease process progresses deeper, eventually localizing in organs that are genetically weak, overused, or already stressed. This is when full-blown disease manifests—diabetes in the pancreas and liver, heart disease in blood vessels, arthritis in joints, skin disorders in blood tissue, or neurological disease in the brain. Ayurveda emphasizes that the organ is not the root cause; it is merely the final victim. The real disease began much earlier with faulty digestion and toxic accumulation.

This Ayurvedic model mirrors modern disease progression remarkably well. Modern science recognizes stages such as insulin resistance before diabetes, fatty liver before cirrhosis, chronic inflammation before autoimmune disease, and gut dysbiosis before mental illness. In all these conditions, functional imbalance precedes structural damage. Ayurveda described this thousands of years ago using different terminology, but the same biological logic. Disease is therefore not an event, but a process.

The greatest strength of this pathophysiological model is its preventive insight. If *Agni* is protected, *Ama* does not form. If *Ama* is prevented, channels remain clear. If channels are clear, tissues remain healthy. And if tissues remain balanced, organs do not fail. This explains why Ayurveda places such emphasis on correct food, proper digestion, meal timing, and compatibility. In simple terms, if waste is not produced in the first place, cleaning and repair become unnecessary. Thus, wrong food creates disease not suddenly, but step by step, through predictable biological failure—making prevention not only possible, but practical and intelligent.

9.5 Preventive Measures – Food Engineering for Health

Preventive health, from both an engineering and biological perspective, begins with controlling the quality of input. No complex system can remain healthy if unsuitable material is repeatedly introduced into it. In the human body, food is the most frequent and powerful input, consumed multiple times every day throughout life. Ayurveda recognized this fundamental truth and emphasized three core principles of healthy eating: *Hitam*, meaning food that is beneficial and supportive of the body; *Ritam*, meaning food consumed at the right time and in harmony with natural biological rhythms; and *Mitam*, meaning food taken in appropriate quantity. These principles are not rigid rules but adaptive guidelines that consider geography, climate, season, age, occupation, digestive strength, and individual constitution.

Hitam food refers to food that the body can easily recognize and utilize. In simple terms, this means fresh, minimally processed, natural foods that provide nourishment without burdening digestion. From engineering science view point, pure fuel in a machine rather than contaminated fuel; the machine runs smoothly with less wear and tear. Similarly, whole grains, fresh vegetables, fruits, natural fats, and properly cooked meals nourish tissues while supporting digestion. Modern nutrition science aligns with this by recommending whole foods rich in fiber, vitamins, minerals, and antioxidants, which support metabolic balance and reduce inflammation.

Ritam emphasizes the importance of timing. Even good food can become harmful if consumed at the wrong time. Eating late at night, skipping meals, or constant snacking disrupts the body's natural digestive rhythm. Ayurveda explains that digestive strength fluctuates during the day, being strongest around midday and weakest at night. A simple example is watering plants at the wrong time of day; excessive watering at night can rot roots, while proper timing promotes growth. Modern science similarly recognizes the importance of circadian rhythms, showing that irregular meal timing disrupts insulin sensitivity, gut function, and hormonal balance.

Mitam focuses on quantity, reminding that overeating is as harmful as poor food quality. Even healthy food, when consumed in excess, overloads digestion and leads to toxic accumulation. A layman's analogy is filling a washing machine beyond capacity; clothes do not get cleaned properly, and the machine suffers damage. Eating according to digestive capacity prevents heaviness, lethargy, and metabolic stress. Modern research supports portion control and mindful eating as key factors in preventing obesity, diabetes, and heart disease.

Daily preventive practices are the practical application of these principles. Avoiding packaged and ultra-processed foods reduces exposure to chemicals, excess sugar, unhealthy fats, and additives. Eating fresh, seasonal meals ensures that food matches environmental conditions and the body's changing needs. Proper hydration supports digestion, circulation, and toxin elimination. Mindful eating—consuming food without screens, stress, or haste—allows the nervous system to activate digestive processes fully. A simple example is eating calmly versus eating while rushing; the same food produces very different digestive outcomes.

Periodic detoxification is another essential aspect of preventive food engineering. Even with good habits, some degree of metabolic waste accumulates over time. Ayurveda recommends practices such as *Langhana* (lightening measures), fasting, and *Panchakarma* to reset digestion and clear accumulated toxins. These practices are not extreme interventions but biological maintenance procedures, similar to periodic servicing of machinery. Modern science supports similar concepts through intermittent fasting, gut reset protocols, and antioxidant replenishment, all of which improve insulin sensitivity, reduce inflammation, and enhance cellular repair.

Repairing damage already done requires patience and systematic correction rather than aggressive suppression of symptoms. Restoring gut microbiota through natural fiber, fermented foods, and reduced chemical exposure improves digestion, immunity, and mental health. Correcting nutritional deficiencies replenishes cellular resources needed for repair. Reducing toxic load by minimizing plastics, pesticides, and additives allows detox organs to recover. Enhancing natural cellular repair mechanisms through adequate sleep, proper nutrition, and stress regulation supports regeneration at the tissue level.

Preventive food engineering ultimately shifts the focus from treating disease to maintaining design integrity. Just as engineers prioritize correct fuel, timing, load, and maintenance to prevent breakdown, human health depends on intelligent food choices practiced consistently. When food quality, timing, and quantity are respected, digestion remains strong, toxins do not accumulate, tissues remain balanced, and organs function optimally. Prevention thus becomes a daily, practical discipline rather than a medical emergency response.

In essence, food engineering for health is not about restriction or fear, but about alignment with biological design. By choosing inputs wisely, the body's inherent intelligence is allowed to function without obstruction. This approach reduces disease risk, slows aging, enhances vitality, and minimizes dependence on medications. True preventive health, therefore, is not achieved through hospitals or laboratories alone, but through conscious, disciplined, and informed food choices made every day.

9.6 Key Take-Home Message

The human body is not a dustbin designed to tolerate unlimited waste; it is a living, intelligent biological masterpiece that responds precisely to what it is repeatedly given. Every cell in the body is built, repaired, and regulated using raw material derived from food. When food quality is natural, compatible, and nourishing, the body maintains balance and resilience. When food is artificial, excessive, or toxic, the same intelligence that once protected health begins to express disease. In simple terms, the body does not randomly fall ill—it faithfully reflects long-term dietary input.

Food should never be viewed as mere calories or stomach-filling material. Every meal carries chemical signals that instruct hormones, immune cells, gut bacteria, and even brain function. Natural foods send clear, coherent instructions that support growth, repair, and stability. Ultra-processed and chemically altered foods send confused or damaging signals, forcing the body into defensive and compensatory modes. A mechanical example is feeding correct software to a computer versus corrupt data; the hardware remains the same, but performance outcomes differ drastically. Similarly, the same body produces health or disease depending on the information it receives through food.

Repeated dietary habits are far more powerful than occasional indulgences. The body can tolerate occasional mistakes, just as a well-maintained machine can handle brief misuse. However, when wrong food becomes routine, damage accumulates silently. Excess sugar programs insulin resistance, unhealthy fats stiffen cell membranes, chemical additives confuse nerve signaling, and toxic residues overload detox pathways. Over the years, these repeated instructions reshape metabolism, immunity, mood, and aging patterns. This explains why chronic diseases develop gradually and often appear "suddenly" only when internal reserves are exhausted.

Food also influences genetic expression through epigenetic mechanisms. While genes themselves may not change, food determines which genes are switched on or off. Poor dietary patterns can activate genes linked to inflammation, obesity, diabetes, and cancer, while nourishing diets promote genes responsible for repair, detoxification, and longevity. A simple analogy is a light switch panel in a house; the wiring is fixed, but which lights remain on depends on daily use. Thus, food choices made today can influence not only present health but also future disease risk.

Preventive health, therefore, does not begin in hospitals, clinics, or pharmacies. These institutions primarily address disease after it has already developed. True prevention begins in kitchens, markets, farms, and daily eating habits. Choosing fresh, seasonal, minimally processed food protects digestion, maintains metabolic balance, and prevents toxic accumulation long before medical intervention is needed. A person who eats intelligently may rarely require medical care, whereas poor dietary habits create lifelong dependence on medications and procedures.

This perspective shifts responsibility and power back to the individual. Health is not solely the outcome of genetics, fate, or medical treatment; it is largely shaped by daily food decisions. Simple practices such as cooking at home, eating mindfully, respecting hunger and fullness, and avoiding unnecessary chemicals act as powerful preventive tools. These practices may appear ordinary, but their long-term impact is profound and cumulative.

Importantly, this message is not meant to promote fear or restriction, but awareness and respect for biological design. Food is meant to nourish, sustain, and strengthen—not to entertain, sedate, or compensate for stress. When food is chosen with understanding rather than impulse, the body's natural intelligence is allowed to function without obstruction. Energy levels improve, immunity strengthens, mental clarity increases, and aging slows naturally.

In summary, the body faithfully mirrors what it is repeatedly fed. Food is instruction, information, and biological programming, not just energy intake. Preventive health is, therefore, a daily practice rooted in conscious eating, not an emergency response after disease appears. When the kitchen becomes the first place of health care, hospitals become places of last resort rather than routine necessity.

9.7 Chapter Summary

This chapter establishes a clear and unavoidable conclusion: unhealthy food is one of the primary drivers of modern disease. The dramatic rise in obesity, diabetes, heart disease, autoimmune disorders, infertility, digestive problems, and mental health conditions cannot be explained by genetics alone. Human biology has remained largely unchanged for thousands of years, while food quality, processing methods, chemical exposure, and eating patterns have changed rapidly within a few generations. This mismatch between biological design and modern dietary input forms the foundation of widespread chronic illness seen today.

A key insight emphasized throughout this chapter is that food-related damage is silent and cumulative. Unlike infections or injuries, unhealthy food does not usually cause immediate symptoms. The body adapts temporarily by overworking digestion, hormones, detoxification systems, and immune defenses. During this adaptive phase, individuals often feel "normal" despite ongoing internal stress. Over time, however, this silent burden exhausts the body's compensatory capacity, and disease emerges suddenly in the form of diabetes, heart attacks, arthritis, liver disease, or mental illness. What appears sudden is, in reality, the final stage of a long, hidden process.

Ayurveda recognized this mechanism of disease development thousands of years ago with remarkable precision. Classical Ayurvedic texts described how wrong food weakens digestion, produces toxic byproducts, blocks bodily channels, and gradually disturbs tissues and organs. These descriptions closely mirror modern scientific concepts such as metabolic dysfunction, chronic inflammation, gut dysbiosis, and cellular toxicity. This convergence demonstrates that traditional wisdom and modern science are not opposing systems, but complementary perspectives describing the same biological reality using different languages.

The chapter also highlights that prevention is not mysterious or complex; it is practical and achievable through intelligent food engineering. Just as engineers protect machines by controlling fuel quality, load, and maintenance schedules, human health can be protected by choosing biologically compatible food, respecting digestion, and minimizing toxic exposure. Simple daily habits—such as eating fresh, seasonal meals, avoiding ultra-processed foods, controlling portion size, and eating mindfully—act as powerful preventive tools. These habits may seem small, but their effects accumulate over time to create lasting health.

Another important message is that medicines, while valuable, have a limited role if input discipline is ignored. Medicines can suppress symptoms, control biochemical parameters, and support recovery during illness, but they cannot override the effects of daily harmful food choices. Treating disease without correcting diet is similar to repairing a machine while continuing to feed it contaminated fuel. Temporary improvement may occur, but relapse or progression is likely. Sustainable healing requires alignment between medical treatment and correct nutritional input.

The chapter also reinforces the concept of personal responsibility in health. While factors such as genetics, environment, and stress influence disease risk, daily food choices remain one of the most controllable determinants of health. Individuals who understand the impact of food on their biology are empowered to prevent disease rather than merely react to it. This understanding transforms health care from a passive dependence on external interventions to an active, informed lifestyle practice.

Importantly, the approach presented is not fear-driven or restrictive. It does not demand perfection or extreme dietary rules. Instead, it promotes awareness, moderation, and consistency. Occasional indulgences do not destroy health; repeated harmful habits do. By focusing on long-term patterns rather than short-term errors, individuals can maintain balance without unnecessary anxiety around food.

In summary, this chapter emphasizes that health is built daily through conscious input, not restored suddenly through emergency intervention. Unhealthy food acts as a slow poison, while appropriate food functions as preventive medicine. When food quality, timing, and quantity are respected, the body's natural intelligence maintains balance and resilience. Thus, true healing and long-term health are not achieved through medicines alone, but through disciplined, informed, and conscious nourishment practiced consistently over a lifetime.

Chapter 10

Longevity Engineering & Rasayana Science

Designing a Long-Life, High-Performance Human System

Longevity is not a mysterious gift granted to a few fortunate individuals; it is the predictable outcome of how the human body is used, fueled, and maintained over long periods of time. Just as engineers design machines with specific limits, maintenance schedules, and fuel requirements, the human body also operates within biological design laws. When these laws are respected, the system runs efficiently for decades; when they are violated, deterioration accelerates. Modern science now confirms that aging is driven by cumulative cellular damage, chronic inflammation, hormonal imbalance, metabolic overload, and declining repair capacity. These processes do not occur overnight. They develop silently through repeated daily habits such as poor diet, irregular sleep, chronic stress, physical inactivity, and neglect of recovery. Therefore, longevity is not accidental; it is the long-term result of disciplined biological engineering.

In everyday life, this concept is easy to understand through simple examples. Consider two houses built in the same year. One is regularly cleaned, repaired, ventilated, and protected from moisture, while the other is ignored, overloaded, and poorly maintained. After twenty or thirty years, the difference between the two is obvious. Cracks, leaks, and decay appear in the neglected house much earlier. The human body behaves in the same way. Cells and tissues are constantly exposed to stress from food, pollution, emotions, workload, and aging itself. If these stresses are balanced with proper nutrition, rest, detoxification, and mental calm, damage is repaired efficiently. If not, wear and tear accumulates, leading to early aging and disease. Thus, long life is the visible outcome of invisible daily maintenance.

Ayurveda described this principle thousands of years ago by stating that life depends on Hitāhita—what is beneficial and what is harmful to the body and mind. According to this view, lifespan is not fixed at birth but is continuously shaped by choices made every day. Eating compatible food strengthens tissues, while incompatible food weakens them. Proper sleep restores nervous and hormonal balance, while sleep deprivation accelerates degeneration. Balanced physical activity maintains circulation and muscle strength, while inactivity leads to stiffness, obesity, and weakness. These ideas align closely with modern findings in preventive medicine, which show that lifestyle-related diseases and premature aging are largely avoidable through consistent healthy behavior.

A clear clinical example can be seen in aging populations. One elderly person may walk independently, think clearly, and remain socially active, while another of the same age may suffer from multiple chronic illnesses, dependence, and mental decline. This difference is often attributed to "luck" or "genes," but deeper examination reveals years of differing habits. The healthier individual typically followed regular routines, ate moderately, managed stress, stayed physically active, and allowed adequate recovery. The weaker individual often lived with chronic stress, irregular meals, excess sugar or fat intake, poor sleep, and neglect of early warning signs. Over time, these small daily differences compound into dramatically different outcomes, proving that longevity is engineered slowly, not decided suddenly.

From an engineering perspective, aging can be understood as a balance between damage and repair. Every day, the body experiences micro-damage at the cellular level due to metabolism, movement, toxins, and stress. Longevity depends on whether the repair systems—digestion, circulation, immunity, sleep, and hormonal regulation—can keep up with this damage. When repair exceeds damage, the body remains youthful and resilient.

When damage exceeds repair, aging accelerates. Ayurveda emphasized strengthening these repair systems through proper diet, daily routines, seasonal adaptation, and rejuvenative therapies. Modern science echoes this through concepts such as cellular repair, antioxidant defense, autophagy, and metabolic health.

In summary, longevity should be understood as a long-term engineering project rather than a short-term medical goal. It is built through thousands of small, consistent actions rather than occasional treatments. Just as a well-maintained vehicle does not break down suddenly, a well-maintained human body does not age rapidly or collapse without warning. True longevity means not merely adding years to life, but adding life to years—maintaining strength, clarity, immunity, and independence. When the body is treated as an intelligent system that requires proper fuel, load management, and regular servicing, a long and healthy life becomes not a matter of chance, but a predictable and achievable outcome.

10.1 Modern Science of Aging: Engineering Failure at the Cellular Level

Modern science now clearly understands aging as a process that begins deep inside the body at the cellular level, long before wrinkles, weakness, or disease become visible. Each cell functions like a self-contained factory with its own power supply, repair units, waste disposal system, and communication network. In youth, these factories run smoothly, repairing daily wear and tear efficiently. With time, however, repeated exposure to poor-quality nutrition, environmental toxins, emotional stress, sleep deprivation, and chronic inflammation slowly damages these systems. Aging, therefore, is not an event that suddenly starts in old age but a gradual decline in cellular efficiency that begins silently in early adulthood and progresses year after year.

One of the most important discoveries in aging research is the identification of the "hallmarks of aging," which are specific types of cellular failures seen across all living organisms. DNA damage is one such failure. DNA acts like an instruction manual or software code for the cell. Every time a cell divides or is exposed to toxins, small errors occur in this code. In a healthy system, repair enzymes correct these errors. With repeated stress and poor repair capacity, mistakes accumulate, leading to malfunctioning cells. A simple example is a photocopy machine that repeatedly copies copies instead of the original; over time, the text becomes faded and distorted. Similarly, repeated uncorrected DNA damage results in aging cells that cannot function optimally.

Another major contributor to aging is telomere shortening. Telomeres are protective caps at the ends of chromosomes, much like the plastic insulation at the end of electrical wires. Each time a cell divides, these caps become slightly shorter. When they become too short, the cell either stops dividing or dies. This is a natural safety mechanism, but chronic stress, poor diet, smoking, obesity, and inflammation accelerate telomere loss. Clinically, this explains why people exposed to long-term stress or unhealthy lifestyles often show signs of premature aging. In simple terms, it is like repeatedly bending a wire until its protective covering wears out, exposing the metal underneath and increasing the risk of breakdown.

Mitochondrial dysfunction is another key feature of cellular aging. Mitochondria are the power plants of the cell, responsible for producing energy. In youth, they generate energy efficiently with minimal waste. With aging, these power plants become damaged and inefficient, producing less energy while releasing more harmful byproducts known as free radicals. This situation is similar to an old generator that gives less electricity but produces more smoke and heat. As a result, tissues with high energy demands—such as the brain, heart, and muscles—are the first to show signs of fatigue, weakness, memory loss, and reduced endurance as aging progresses.

Chronic low-grade inflammation, often referred to as "inflammaging," is another central mechanism of aging. Inflammation is meant to be a short-term repair response, like a fire alarm that activates only during emergencies. When poor lifestyle habits keep this alarm switched on continuously, it damages healthy tissues. Constant inflammation slowly destroys joints, blood vessels, nerves, and organs, accelerating aging and increasing the risk of diseases such as diabetes, heart disease, arthritis, and neurodegeneration. A layman's comparison would be a machine that constantly runs at high temperature; even if it continues working, its internal parts wear out much faster than a machine that operates within safe limits.

Importantly, modern science emphasizes that these cellular failures are not fixed or irreversible in their early stages. Aging speed is influenced by how well the body's repair and maintenance systems function. Proper nutrition supplies raw materials for repair, sleep activates cellular cleanup and regeneration, physical activity improves mitochondrial efficiency, and stress control reduces inflammatory damage. This understanding aligns with the engineering principle of preventive maintenance. Just as early servicing can extend the life of a machine, reducing cellular stress early in life can significantly slow biological aging. Therefore, aging should be viewed not as an unavoidable countdown, but as a modifiable process that responds to intelligent, timely intervention at the cellular level.

10.2 Ayurvedic Concept of Longevity: Ayushya and Rasayana

Ayurveda defines longevity through the concept of **Ayushya,** which means not just the length of life but the quality and usefulness of that life. A long lifespan without strength, clarity, digestion, immunity, or emotional balance is not considered true longevity in Ayurveda. Classical Ayurvedic thought emphasizes that the purpose of living longer is to remain capable, independent, mentally alert, and socially functional. From this perspective, aging is acceptable, but degeneration is not. Longevity is therefore measured by how well the body maintains its functional intelligence over time rather than by the number of years survived.

Central to this understanding is the concept of **Rasayana,** a specialized branch of Ayurveda dedicated to rejuvenation, tissue nourishment, and resistance against aging and disease. Rasayana literally means "the path that nourishes rasa," where *rasa* represents the primary nourishing fluid that ultimately sustains all tissues of the body. If nourishment is weak at this foundational level, every subsequent tissue—blood, muscle, fat, bone, nerve, and reproductive tissue—becomes progressively weaker. Rasayana therapies are designed to improve this foundational nourishment so that every tissue receives adequate, high-quality nutrition and maintains its structure and function for a longer time.

A simple layman's analogy can clarify this concept. Imagine a city supplied by a central water system. Even if plenty of water is available, damaged pipelines, blockages, or leakage will prevent proper distribution to homes. Similarly, eating nutritious food alone does not guarantee vitality if digestion is weak, circulation is poor, or metabolic waste is accumulated. Rasayana works like repairing pipelines, cleaning blockages, and strengthening the distribution system so that nourishment reaches every cell efficiently. This is why Rasayana is not just about adding supplements but about improving digestion, metabolism, circulation, and cellular uptake.

Ayurveda also recognizes that aging accelerates when the body's internal environment becomes hostile to repair. Poor digestion leads to toxic byproducts, disturbed sleep weakens nervous regulation, chronic stress exhausts hormonal balance, and unresolved inflammation damages tissues. Rasayana corrects this internal environment by calming the nervous system, stabilizing digestion, enhancing immunity, and supporting tissue regeneration. For example, a person with a good appetite but poor absorption may feel weak despite eating well. Rasayana therapies aim to correct this inefficiency so that strength, immunity, and endurance gradually improve rather than decline with age.

Another important aspect of Rasayana is its effect on mental and emotional longevity. Ayurveda clearly states that clarity of mind, emotional stability, memory, and enthusiasm are essential components of long life. Chronic anxiety, fear, anger, and grief accelerate aging just as surely as poor diet or lack of sleep. Rasayana includes lifestyle discipline, mental regulation, ethical conduct, and adequate rest to preserve mental balance. In simple terms, a calm and content mind allows the body to repair itself efficiently, while a constantly disturbed mind keeps the body in a state of internal stress and breakdown.

Importantly, Rasayana is not a short-term treatment given after disease appears; it is a long-term biological optimization strategy. It is most effective when used preventively or during early stages of decline. Just as reinforcing a bridge before cracks appear is more effective than repairing it after collapse, strengthening tissues and repair mechanisms early in life preserves function for decades. Ayurveda therefore recommends Rasayana after detoxification, during seasonal transitions, and at specific stages of life to slow degeneration and enhance resilience.

In summary, the Ayurvedic concept of longevity views the human body as a living system that must be continuously optimized, not merely repaired after failure. Ayushya is achieved when nourishment is efficient, repair is timely, waste is removed, and the mind remains balanced. Rasayana serves as the engineering protocol that maintains this balance. By strengthening the internal environment, improving tissue quality, and supporting mental clarity, Rasayana allows nutrition, rest, and lifestyle discipline to truly translate into lasting vitality. Thus, Ayurveda presents longevity not as a miracle or destiny, but as the predictable outcome of intelligent, sustained biological care.

10.3 Longevity Engineering: Correlating Ayurveda and Modern Science

Longevity engineering becomes most convincing when the principles of Ayurveda and modern biomedical science are placed side by side. Although they use different languages and conceptual frameworks, both systems ultimately describe the same biological realities. Modern longevity research explains aging in terms of oxidative stress, mitochondrial inefficiency, chronic inflammation, hormonal dysregulation, and declining cellular repair. Ayurveda explains the same decline through weakened digestion (*Agni*), improper tissue nourishment (*Dhatu poshana*), reduced vitality (*Ojas*), and disturbed mental balance. When these descriptions are carefully compared, it becomes clear that Rasayana is not a mystical idea but an early, holistic model of biological maintenance and repair.

One of the clearest correlations lies in the concept of digestion and metabolism. Modern science recognizes that excess calories, poor-quality food, and irregular eating overload metabolic pathways, leading to insulin resistance, fat accumulation, inflammation, and accelerated aging. Ayurveda described this exact problem thousands of years ago, warning that overeating, incompatible food combinations, and eating without proper hunger weaken *Agni*, the digestive fire. When digestion is weak, nourishment is incomplete and toxic byproducts accumulate. In simple terms, this is like overloading a furnace with low-quality fuel; instead of producing steady heat, it generates smoke and residue that damage the system. Both sciences agree that controlled intake, proper timing of meals, and digestive efficiency are foundational to long life.

Another strong overlap is seen in the understanding of cellular energy and mitochondrial health. Modern science identifies mitochondria as key regulators of aging, noting that inefficient energy production leads to fatigue, organ decline, and increased oxidative damage. Ayurveda addresses this through the concept of strong *Dhatus*, especially muscle, nerve, and reproductive tissues, which depend on efficient energy conversion. Rasayana therapies aim to improve energy utilization at the tissue level, ensuring that nourishment is not wasted but converted into strength and endurance. A simple example would be upgrading an engine so that it extracts maximum mileage from the same amount of fuel, rather than burning fuel inefficiently and producing excess exhaust.

Chronic inflammation is another area where both systems align closely. Modern medicine describes "inflammaging," a state of persistent low-grade inflammation that slowly damages organs and accelerates aging. Ayurveda describes a similar state through the accumulation of *Ama*, a toxic residue formed when digestion and metabolism are incomplete. This *Ama* circulates through the body, blocking channels and irritating tissues, leading to joint pain, fatigue, poor immunity, and early degeneration. From an engineering perspective, this is like sludge accumulating in pipelines, reducing flow and increasing internal pressure. Rasayana, especially when preceded by detoxification, focuses on clearing these blockages so that tissues remain clean, flexible, and responsive.

The role of mental and emotional health provides another powerful point of convergence. Modern research shows that chronic psychological stress increases cortisol levels, damages mitochondria, suppresses immunity, and shortens telomeres, thereby accelerating biological aging. Ayurveda emphasized mental discipline, emotional balance, and calmness as essential pillars of long life. Excessive fear, anger, grief, or anxiety were considered direct causes of tissue depletion and loss of vitality. In simple terms, a constantly stressed mind keeps the body in emergency mode, diverting energy away from repair and regeneration. Both systems, therefore, agree that mental stability is not optional for longevity; it is a biological necessity.

Modern longevity science also highlights the importance of activating repair pathways such as cellular cleanup, regeneration, and adaptive stress responses. Practices like intermittent fasting, exercise, and adequate sleep are now known to stimulate these pathways. Ayurveda incorporated similar principles through daily routines, seasonal adaptation, moderation in food, physical activity, and restorative sleep. Rasayana strengthens these natural repair processes rather than forcing artificial stimulation. It works by improving the body's internal intelligence so that repair happens continuously and efficiently, much like a self-monitoring machine that detects wear early and corrects it automatically.

In conclusion, longevity engineering represents the meeting point of ancient wisdom and modern science. Ayurveda provided a system-level understanding of how digestion, nourishment, immunity, and mental balance determine the speed of aging. Modern science has validated these insights at the cellular and molecular level. Rasayana emerges as a comprehensive maintenance protocol that reduces stress on the system, enhances repair capacity, and preserves functional integrity. This convergence clearly demonstrates that true longevity is not achieved through isolated interventions but through sustained, intelligent management of the human biological system over time.

10.4 Rasayana Therapy: Types and Engineering Logic

Rasayana therapy in Ayurveda is designed with a clear engineering logic that recognizes different levels of wear, damage, and repair needs in the human body. Just as machines are not maintained by a single method, the body also requires different rejuvenation strategies depending on age, strength, disease burden, and lifestyle. Ayurveda, therefore, classified Rasayana into different types, primarily **Kutipraveshika Rasayana** and **Vatatapika Rasayana,** to match the intensity of intervention with the condition of the system. This classification reflects a sophisticated understanding that deep repair requires controlled conditions, while long-term preservation requires regular, sustainable maintenance.

Kutipraveshika Rasayana represents the most intensive form of rejuvenation therapy. It is conducted in a specially prepared, controlled environment where exposure to wind, sun, noise, stress, and external disturbances is minimized. The individual follows strict dietary rules, regulated daily routines, mental discipline, and carefully selected rejuvenative formulations. From an engineering perspective, this is equivalent to a complete system shutdown and overhaul. A machine undergoing major refurbishment is removed from regular operation, dismantled, cleaned, repaired, and reassembled under expert supervision. Similarly, Kutipraveshika Rasayana allows the body's repair mechanisms to operate without interference from external stressors, leading to deep tissue rejuvenation, improved immunity, sharper mental function, and noticeable slowing of aging processes.

To understand this in simple layman's terms, consider a severely worn vehicle that has been running continuously for years. Quick servicing will not restore its performance. It needs to be taken off the road, stripped down, and rebuilt. Kutipraveshika Rasayana serves this role in humans who show significant degeneration, premature aging, or chronic depletion. Because this process demands isolation, discipline, and time, it is not practical for everyone, but when performed correctly, it produces profound and long-lasting benefits by resetting the body's internal balance and repair capacity.

Vatatapika Rasayana, in contrast, is designed for individuals living active, everyday lives. It does not require isolation or extreme environmental control. Instead, it integrates rejuvenation into daily routine through appropriate diet, lifestyle discipline, seasonal adaptation, and regular use of Rasayana formulations. This approach is comparable to routine servicing of a well-functioning machine. Oil changes, lubrication, filter cleaning, and minor adjustments may seem small, but they prevent friction, overheating, and sudden failure. Over time, such maintenance significantly extends the life and efficiency of the system.

In practical terms, Vatatapika Rasayana is ideal for working professionals, elderly individuals maintaining independence, and even younger people aiming to prevent early aging. A person who eats moderately, sleeps regularly, manages stress, and uses rejuvenative support maintains steady energy, clear digestion, and stronger immunity. Although the changes may be gradual, they accumulate over the years to produce remarkable resilience. This explains why Ayurveda emphasizes consistency over intensity for long-term health, recognizing that small daily corrections prevent the need for major repair later.

Importantly, both Kutipraveshika and Vatatapika Rasayana serve the same fundamental goal: slowing degeneration and enhancing repair. The difference lies in timing, intensity, and feasibility. Kutipraveshika is corrective and restorative, suitable when damage is advanced. Vatatapika is preventive and preservative, suitable for ongoing life. Together, they form a complete longevity engineering framework that mirrors modern maintenance science—major overhaul when required, and continuous servicing to prevent breakdown.

In summary, Rasayana therapy is not a single medicine or isolated treatment, but a strategic system of biological engineering. Ayurveda recognized that longevity depends on matching the level of intervention to the condition of the body. Whether through intensive rejuvenation in controlled settings or steady maintenance within daily life, Rasayana works by reducing wear, improving repair efficiency, and preserving functional integrity. This logical, engineering-based approach explains why Rasayana remains one of the most advanced longevity models ever described, fully relevant even in the age of modern biomedical science.

10.5 Important Rasayana Drugs and Their Scientific Correlates

Rasayana drugs occupy a unique position in Ayurveda because they are not designed for short-term symptom relief but for long-term optimization of the body's internal environment. Their primary role is to enhance resilience, repair capacity, and regulation rather than forcing artificial stimulation. Modern science now describes similar substances as adaptogens, antioxidants, immunomodulators, and neuroprotective agents. Although the terminology differs, the underlying biological logic is remarkably similar. These Rasayana substances act like intelligent engineering upgrades that strengthen weak points in the system so that daily stress and aging do not translate into progressive damage.

Ashwagandha is one of the most widely studied Rasayana herbs and is best understood as a stress-buffering agent. Chronic stress keeps the body in a constant state of alarm, raising cortisol levels and slowly damaging muscles, nerves, digestion, and immunity. Ashwagandha helps normalize this stress response rather than suppressing it completely. A simple analogy is a shock absorber in a vehicle. Without it, every bump on the road directly damages the vehicle's structure. With a good shock absorber, the same bumps are absorbed, and long-term damage is prevented. Similarly, Ashwagandha allows the body to face stress without allowing stress to erode tissue strength and vitality over time.

Amalaki plays a central role in Rasayana therapy due to its powerful antioxidant and metabolic-regulating properties. Oxidative stress is a major driver of cellular aging, comparable to rust slowly corroding metal parts of a machine. Amalaki acts like an internal rust-prevention system by neutralizing free radicals and supporting efficient metabolism. From a practical perspective, this explains why Amalaki supports skin health, digestion, immunity, and overall energy. A person consuming nutritious food may still age rapidly if oxidative damage is high; Amalaki helps preserve the quality of tissues so that nourishment is not wasted through ongoing cellular injury.

Guduchi is valued for its role in strengthening immune intelligence rather than merely boosting immune activity. Modern medicine recognizes that many age-related diseases arise from immune imbalance—either weak responses that allow infections or excessive responses that cause chronic inflammation and autoimmune disorders. Guduchi helps regulate this balance. In common man's terms, it works like a well-trained security system that identifies real threats accurately without sounding false alarms. By improving discrimination and regulation, Guduchi reduces unnecessary inflammation while preserving the body's ability to defend itself, which is crucial for long-term health and longevity.

Herbs such as Brahmi and Mandukaparni are classic examples of Rasayana substances that focus on the nervous system. The brain and nerves are among the most delicate and energy-demanding tissues in the body, making them especially vulnerable to aging, stress, and oxidative damage. These herbs support memory, concentration, emotional stability, and sleep quality. A useful analogy is insulation around electrical wiring. Without proper insulation, signals leak, circuits malfunction, and breakdowns occur. Brahmi and Mandukaparni act like protective insulation for neural circuits, ensuring efficient signal transmission and reducing wear caused by chronic mental stress.

An important engineering principle behind Rasayana drugs is that they do not override the body's intelligence. Unlike stimulants that force energy output at the cost of future exhaustion, Rasayana substances enhance the body's inherent regulatory systems. They improve digestion so nourishment is properly absorbed, support circulation so nutrients reach tissues, stabilize the nervous system so repair can occur, and balance immunity so damage is minimized. This explains why their effects are gradual but sustained, much like reinforcing the foundation of a building rather than repeatedly repairing cracks on the surface.

In combination, these Rasayana drugs function as a coordinated maintenance system. Ashwagandha protects against stress-induced wear, Amalaki guards against oxidative corrosion, Guduchi ensures immune balance, and Brahmi and Mandukaparni preserve cognitive and emotional stability. Together, they support the core pillars of longevity—energy, immunity, mental clarity, and tissue integrity. This integrated action demonstrates that Rasayana therapy is not about forcing youthfulness but about preserving biological order and efficiency. By enhancing natural repair and regulation, these substances help the body age slowly, gracefully, and with functional independence, which is the true goal of longevity engineering.

10.6 Panchakarma Before Rasayana: The Engineering Necessity

Ayurveda places strong emphasis on performing Panchakarma before Rasayana because true rejuvenation is impossible without prior cleansing. This principle follows clear engineering logic. If a system is clogged with waste, corrosion, or sludge, adding superior fuel or lubricants will not improve performance; instead, it may push contaminants deeper into critical components. Similarly, the human body accumulates metabolic waste, inflammatory byproducts, and undigested residues over years of improper diet, stress, poor sleep, and illness. Rasayana therapies are designed to nourish and rebuild tissues, but if the internal environment is polluted, nourishment cannot be properly absorbed or utilized. Panchakarma, therefore, prepares the biological system so that rejuvenation can occur efficiently and safely.

From a layman's perspective, this can be understood by considering soil and fertilizer. Even the best fertilizer will fail if the soil is compacted, toxic, or waterlogged. The first step must be clearing debris, aerating the soil, and restoring its natural structure. Panchakarma performs this role inside the body. By cleansing the digestive tract, circulation pathways, and tissue channels, it restores the body's ability to receive and distribute nourishment. Once this internal terrain is corrected, Rasayana therapies can truly strengthen tissues, immunity, and vitality rather than producing superficial or short-lived benefits.

Ayurveda explains this process through the removal of *Ama*, which represents toxic, sticky metabolic waste formed due to weak digestion and improper metabolism. *Ama* obstructs channels (*Srotas*), disrupts tissue nourishment, and fuels chronic inflammation. Clinically, this manifests as fatigue, heaviness, joint stiffness, poor appetite, skin disorders, and recurrent illness. Panchakarma procedures reduce this burden, allowing digestion (*Agni*) to reset and circulation to normalize. In simple terms, this is similar to flushing blocked pipes before increasing water pressure; without clearing blockages, increased flow only worsens leaks and damage.

Modern science offers a parallel explanation through the concept of cellular cleanup and recycling. Processes such as autophagy remove damaged proteins, dysfunctional mitochondria, and cellular debris before new components are synthesized. When this cleanup is impaired, damaged structures accumulate, accelerating aging and disease. Panchakarma mirrors this principle at the systemic level. By reducing inflammatory load, oxidative stress, and metabolic congestion, it creates conditions in which the body's natural repair mechanisms can function optimally. Without this preparatory phase, attempts at rejuvenation resemble building new machinery on a foundation filled with debris.

Another important aspect is inflammation control. Chronic low-grade inflammation keeps the body in a constant state of repair emergency, diverting energy away from regeneration and longevity. Rasayana aims to strengthen tissues and immunity, but if inflammation is already high, the body prioritizes defense over rebuilding. Panchakarma reduces this background inflammatory noise, allowing the body to shift from survival mode to regeneration mode. A simple analogy is trying to renovate a building while a fire alarm is constantly ringing; meaningful work cannot proceed until the emergency is resolved.

Panchakarma also improves digestive efficiency, which is critical for Rasayana success. Rejuvenative substances rely on proper digestion and absorption to reach tissues. If digestion is weak, even the finest Rasayana formulations remain underutilized or may contribute to further metabolic burden. Cleansing therapies restore appetite, improve gut function, and enhance nutrient assimilation. This is similar to calibrating a machine before installing high-performance components; without proper calibration, upgrades fail to deliver expected results.

In summary, Panchakarma before Rasayana is not a ritualistic sequence but a rational engineering requirement. Cleansing removes obstacles, resets regulatory systems, and lowers internal stress, creating a receptive biological environment. Rasayana then builds upon this clean foundation to strengthen tissues, immunity, and mental clarity. Without detoxification, rejuvenation remains partial and temporary; with proper cleansing, repair becomes deeper, more efficient, and longer lasting. This sequential approach reflects a profound understanding of system maintenance—clean first, then rebuild—which remains as relevant today as it was in classical Ayurveda.

10.7 Lifestyle Rasayana: Achar Rasayana

Ayurveda clearly states that medicines alone cannot secure long life if daily behavior continuously damages the body and mind. This understanding is expressed through **Achar Rasayana**, the code of conduct and lifestyle discipline meant to preserve longevity. Achar Rasayana focuses on how a person thinks, reacts, rests, communicates, and lives in society. These factors directly influence the nervous system, hormonal balance, immunity, and digestion. From an engineering viewpoint, this is equivalent to maintaining a stable operating system. Even the best hardware fails quickly if the software is unstable, overloaded, or infected with errors. Similarly, a disturbed lifestyle undermines all physical rejuvenation efforts.

One of the most important elements of Achar Rasayana is emotional regulation. Ayurveda recognized that uncontrolled anger, fear, anxiety, jealousy, and grief steadily deplete vitality. Modern science confirms that chronic emotional stress keeps stress hormones elevated, disrupts sleep, suppresses immunity, and accelerates cellular aging. In simple terms, a body under constant emotional strain behaves like a machine that is never switched off. Even if it continues to function, internal components wear out much faster. Emotional balance allows the body to enter repair mode regularly, which is essential for long-term health and slow aging.

Adequate rest and sleep are another cornerstone of lifestyle Rasayana. Ayurveda emphasized proper timing and quality of sleep as a non-negotiable requirement for longevity. Today, research shows that deep sleep activates cellular repair, hormonal regulation, immune renewal, and brain detoxification. A person who eats well but sleeps poorly often ages faster than someone with an average diet but consistent restorative sleep. This can be easily understood by comparing two smartphones with identical batteries: one is charged fully every night, while the other is repeatedly used until empty and charged irregularly. Over time, battery health declines much faster in the poorly managed device.

Social behavior and ethical conduct also play a significant role in Achar Rasayana. Truthfulness, respect, compassion, and harmonious relationships reduce internal psychological conflict. Constant guilt, deception, hostility, or social isolation creates persistent mental stress, even if the individual appears outwardly successful. Ayurveda understood that inner conflict generates continuous stress signals that disturb digestion, circulation, and immunity. In layman's terms, it is like driving a vehicle with the handbrake partially engaged. The engine works harder, fuel efficiency drops, and parts wear out faster—even though the vehicle appears to be moving normally.

Mindfulness and self-awareness form another essential aspect of lifestyle Rasayana. Being aware of one's limits, hunger, fatigue, and emotional state prevents overload. Modern neuroscience shows that mindful awareness activates calming neural pathways and improves stress resilience. Ayurveda encouraged conscious living—eating when hungry, resting when tired, and responding thoughtfully rather than impulsively. This is similar to a smart control system that senses overload early and adjusts performance before damage occurs. A person lacking such awareness often ignores early warning signs, pushing the body until breakdown occurs.

A powerful illustration of Achar Rasayana can be seen in two individuals with similar diet and physical health. One lives with constant deadlines, poor sleep, emotional tension, and little mental rest. The other maintains regular sleep, emotional balance, meaningful relationships, and calm routines. Over the years, the first individual often develops premature aging, metabolic disorders, or immune problems, while the second remains stable and energetic. This difference arises not from food or medicine, but from lifestyle intelligence. Ayurveda recognized this long before modern stress biology existed.

In summary, Achar Rasayana forms the foundation of all longevity strategies. Medicines, detoxification, and nutrition can enhance health, but without behavioral and mental discipline, their benefits remain limited and temporary. Lifestyle Rasayana protects the nervous and hormonal systems, reduces internal wear, and allows the body's natural repair mechanisms to function consistently. By acting as a stable operating system for the human body, Achar Rasayana ensures that longevity is not just extended in years, but preserved in strength, clarity, and functional independence.

10.8 Integrated Longevity Engineering Model

Longevity should be understood as the outcome of an integrated biological system rather than the result of any single medicine, therapy, or lifestyle habit. The human body functions through multiple interdependent subsystems—nutrition, digestion, metabolism, detoxification, immunity, nervous regulation, and tissue repair. Each of these systems supports the others, and failure in one gradually burdens the rest. Just as complex engineering systems like aircraft or power plants rely on the coordinated performance of many components, the human body requires synchronized functioning to sustain long life. Longevity emerges when all systems operate within safe limits and support one another continuously.

Food is the starting point of this integrated model because it provides the raw material and fuel for every biological process. However, food alone does not create health. Efficient digestion is required to convert food into usable energy and building blocks. A person may consume nutritious meals, yet still feel weak or unhealthy if digestion is impaired. This is similar to filling a fuel tank with high-quality fuel while the engine's combustion system is faulty; fuel is present, but energy output remains poor. Ayurveda and modern science both emphasize that digestion determines whether nourishment becomes strength or waste.

Detoxification plays an equally important role in maintaining system efficiency. Daily metabolism produces waste, and improper digestion adds further toxic burden. If this waste is not cleared, it obstructs pathways, irritates tissues, and triggers inflammation. In engineering terms, this resembles debris accumulating in pipes and filters. Even if fuel quality is excellent, blocked channels reduce efficiency and increase pressure on the system. Periodic detoxification ensures that circulation, metabolism, and cellular communication remain clear, allowing nutrients and oxygen to reach every tissue effectively.

Immunity and repair mechanisms act as the system's protective and maintenance units. The immune system identifies threats and manages damage, while repair mechanisms restore worn tissues. When immunity is weak, infections and degeneration increase; when immunity is excessive or misdirected, chronic inflammation and autoimmune damage occur. Both scenarios accelerate aging. This balance mirrors security and maintenance teams in high-value systems, which must be vigilant but not overreactive. Proper immunity preserves longevity by preventing damage without creating unnecessary internal conflict.

Mental balance and nervous system regulation form the control center of the longevity model. Chronic stress continuously signals danger, diverting energy away from digestion, repair, and regeneration toward survival responses. Over time, this leads to hormonal imbalance, immune suppression, and faster aging. A calm, regulated nervous system allows the body to shift regularly into repair mode. In simple terms, a machine constantly running at emergency speed wears out faster than one that alternates intelligently between work and rest. Emotional stability, adequate sleep, and mindful living are therefore not optional luxuries but core components of longevity engineering.

Rasayana therapy fits into this integrated model as periodic system renewal rather than daily fuel or routine servicing. Even well-maintained systems experience gradual wear over time. Rasayana restores declining reserves, improves tissue quality, and enhances resilience, much like scheduled overhauls in long-running machines. However, Rasayana cannot compensate for poor fuel, blocked pathways, weak digestion, or chronic stress. Its effectiveness depends on the health of the supporting systems, reinforcing the idea that no single intervention can override systemic neglect.

A common example illustrates this integration clearly. Consider two individuals taking the same rejuvenative medicine. One eats irregularly, sleeps poorly, lives under constant stress, and ignores digestion. The other eats moderately, sleeps well, manages emotions, and maintains routine cleansing. Over time, the second individual experiences sustained energy and slower aging, while the first sees minimal benefit. The difference lies not in the medicine but in the supporting systems that allow the medicine to work.

In summary, integrated longevity engineering recognizes that the human body is a complex, self-regulating system requiring continuous, coordinated care. Food, digestion, detoxification, immunity, mental balance, sleep, and rejuvenation must function together like interconnected subsystems of a high-value machine. Ignoring even one element places excessive load on the others, accelerating failure. True longevity is therefore achieved not through isolated excellence, but through balanced, intelligent maintenance of the entire human system over a lifetime.

10.9 Future of Longevity: Preventive, Not Reactive

The future of longevity is increasingly understood as preventive engineering rather than reactive repair. For decades, healthcare systems focused mainly on diagnosing and treating disease after symptoms became obvious. By that stage, significant damage had already occurred at the cellular, metabolic, or organ level. Modern science is now recognizing that this approach is inefficient, costly, and often incapable of restoring full function. As a result, attention is shifting toward predictive biomarkers, early risk detection, personalized nutrition, and lifestyle-based prevention. This shift closely mirrors the Ayurvedic philosophy that health must be protected continuously, long before disease announces itself.

Predictive medicine aims to identify early warning signals—such as metabolic imbalance, inflammation markers, hormonal disruption, or genetic susceptibility—before illness develops. Ayurveda described similar early warning stages through subtle changes in digestion, energy, sleep, mood, and elimination. These signs were not ignored but used to guide corrective action. In simple terms, this is like detecting unusual vibrations or temperature changes in a machine before a major breakdown occurs. Acting early allows small corrections to prevent large failures, preserving both function and longevity.

Personalization is another defining feature of future longevity care. Modern research increasingly shows that the same diet, exercise plan, or supplement does not suit everyone equally. Ayurveda addressed this centuries ago by tailoring lifestyle, food, and routines according to individual constitution, age, season, and environment. An example makes this clear: two people may eat the same food, yet one digests it easily while the other develops discomfort or disease. The difference lies in individual capacity, not the food alone. The future of healthcare recognizes this reality and moves away from one-size-fits-all solutions toward individualized health engineering.

Preventive longevity also emphasizes maintaining function rather than merely prolonging survival. Living longer while dependent, fatigued, or cognitively impaired is not considered success. Both modern longevity science and Ayurveda now converge on the idea that true long life must preserve strength, mobility, immunity, mental clarity, and emotional stability. This is similar to maintaining a high-performance system that continues to operate smoothly over time rather than barely functioning until final failure. Longevity, in this sense, is about sustained performance, not delayed collapse.

Another important shift in future healthcare is the focus on integrating lifestyle, nutrition, mental health, and periodic rejuvenation rather than relying solely on pharmaceuticals. Medicines are valuable tools, but they are most effective when the underlying system is balanced. Ayurveda always placed primary emphasis on daily routine, seasonal adaptation, stress regulation, and timely rejuvenation. Modern science now supports this approach by demonstrating that sleep, movement, emotional balance, and diet directly influence gene expression, immune function, and aging speed. This reinforces the idea that health is engineered daily, not rescued occasionally.

A simple comparison highlights this preventive mindset. Consider two individuals with similar genetic risk for chronic disease. One waits for symptoms and seeks treatment only after diagnosis. The other monitors health parameters, adapts lifestyle early, manages stress, and undergoes periodic maintenance. Over decades, the second individual often avoids major illness altogether or experiences milder, delayed disease. The difference is not luck, but proactive design. Preventive action changes the trajectory of aging long before a crisis appears.

In conclusion, the future of longevity lies in respecting the human body as an intelligently designed biological system with predictable rules of operation. When these rules are understood and followed, health becomes stable and disease becomes less likely. Ayurveda provided this preventive blueprint long ago, and modern science is now validating it through advanced tools and measurements. Longevity, therefore, is not about fighting death after disease has taken hold, but about engineering life so efficiently that disease struggles to arise. When health is maintained intelligently and consistently, long life becomes a logical, achievable outcome rather than a fortunate accident.

10.10 Closing Note

Longevity should be understood as the cumulative outcome of countless small, intelligent choices rather than the effect of a single intervention. No medicine, supplement, genetic trait, or advanced technology can override years of biological neglect. Just as a well-designed system performs reliably only when it is operated within limits and maintained regularly, the human body responds predictably to how it is treated over time. Health and long life emerge when nutrition, digestion, rest, movement, emotional balance, and recovery are aligned consistently. When these fundamentals are ignored, even the most advanced therapies can offer only temporary relief, not lasting vitality.

A common misunderstanding about longevity is the idea that living longer automatically means living better. In reality, adding years without strength, clarity, or independence often increases suffering rather than fulfillment. Ayurveda and modern longevity science both emphasize that the goal is not merely survival, but functional life—being able to think clearly, move independently, digest comfortably, and engage meaningfully with society. A person who lives to an advanced age but remains dependent and chronically ill has technically extended life, but has not achieved true longevity. True longevity preserves dignity, usefulness, and quality of experience.

This distinction becomes clear through simple everyday examples. Consider two individuals of the same age. One maintained regular routines, moderate eating habits, emotional balance, and periodic rest throughout life. The other lived with chronic stress, irregular meals, poor sleep, and neglect of early health signals. In later years, the first individual often remains active and mentally sharp, while the second struggles with multiple illnesses and dependence. The difference is not a miracle or coincidence; it is the visible result of long-term biological management versus long-term overload.

Longevity engineering works on the principle of accumulation. Small daily actions—such as sleeping on time, eating according to hunger, managing emotions, and allowing recovery—may seem insignificant in isolation. However, over decades, these actions compound into resilience and strength.

This is similar to saving money regularly. Small, consistent deposits create financial security over time, while sporadic large deposits cannot compensate for years of neglect. In the same way, consistent health-supporting habits build a reserve of vitality that protects against aging-related decline.

Another important aspect of intelligent longevity is respecting the body's warning signals. Fatigue, indigestion, irritability, poor sleep, and recurring minor illnesses are not inconveniences to be suppressed; they are early indicators of imbalance. Ignoring them is equivalent to ignoring warning lights on a dashboard. Responding early with rest, dietary correction, stress reduction, or detoxification prevents deeper damage. This approach transforms healthcare from crisis management into continuous optimization, which is far more effective and humane.

As people age, the goal of longevity shifts from growth to preservation and wisdom. When the body is well maintained, aging becomes a phase of refinement rather than decline. Energy may be used more selectively, but clarity, experience, and emotional stability often increase. Such aging allows individuals to contribute meaningfully to family and society rather than becoming burdensome. This is why Ayurveda viewed long life as valuable only when accompanied by mental clarity, ethical conduct, and social harmony.

In conclusion, longevity is not a miracle to be discovered but a system to be managed. It rewards those who apply intelligent biological engineering consistently over time. Adding years without vitality serves little purpose, but adding vitality to years transforms aging into a period of strength, insight, and dignity. When the human body is respected as a finely tuned biological system and cared for accordingly, long life ceases to be an accident and becomes a natural, logical outcome of how life is lived.

Chapter 11

Artificial Intelligence Vs Human Body Intelligence

11.1 A Comparative Engineering Analysis

Artificial intelligence is often presented as the highest form of intelligence created by humans, yet this perception arises largely from misunderstanding what intelligence truly means in a biological sense. Artificial intelligence operates only within the narrow boundaries of what it is programmed or trained to do. It processes data, recognizes patterns, and generates outputs based on mathematical rules, but it has no understanding of meaning, no awareness of context beyond data correlations, no capacity for self-preservation, and no intrinsic purpose. It is comparable to a very fast calculator or an extremely advanced spreadsheet — powerful, but fundamentally blind to life. The human body, on the other hand, is not merely intelligent in one domain; it is intelligent across physical, chemical, emotional, cognitive, immune, hormonal, and regenerative domains simultaneously. It does not need external commands to function; it continuously senses, decides, adapts, and corrects itself moment by moment.

From an engineering perspective, artificial intelligence is a *single-function tool*, while the human body is a *multi-layered autonomous system.* AI depends entirely on electricity, hardware stability, data quality, and human supervision. If any of these fail, the system stops or produces errors. The human body, however, functions continuously without shutdowns, maintenance engineers, or software updates. It repairs its own tissues, replaces damaged cells, defends itself against infections, regulates temperature, balances fluids and electrolytes, detoxifies waste, adapts metabolism to food availability, and adjusts emotional and mental states according to environmental and social conditions — all without conscious instruction. A example is that a smartphone needs charging, servicing, and updates, while a human child grows, heals wounds, learns language, builds immunity, and adapts to the climate without anyone programming these processes into them.

Artificial intelligence does not possess self-awareness, subjective experience, or internal values. It does not know that it exists, it does not feel hunger, pain, fear, love, fatigue, or motivation, and it has no concept of survival or well-being. The human body's intelligence, however, is deeply rooted in survival logic and self-preservation. Hunger guides nutrition, pain signals injury, fear triggers protection, pleasure reinforces beneficial behavior, and fatigue enforces rest and repair. These are not emotions in isolation; they are biological feedback signals designed to preserve system integrity. A example is that if you touch a hot surface, you instantly withdraw your hand without thinking, protecting yourself automatically. No artificial system withdraws itself from damage unless explicitly programmed and connected to sensors and logic for that specific case.

Another major difference lies in adaptability and learning. Artificial intelligence can only learn within the limits of the data it receives and the structure of its model. It cannot redefine its own goals, create new purposes, or reorganize itself fundamentally. The human body, however, continuously reprograms itself through epigenetics, neuroplasticity, immune memory, hormonal adaptation, and metabolic adjustment. If a person moves to a cold climate, their circulation, metabolism, and even fat distribution adapt over time. If a person practices a new skill, the brain physically rewires itself to support it. If a person is exposed to a new pathogen, the immune system learns and remembers it for decades.

This capacity for self-restructuring without external engineering is unmatched by any artificial system.

Artificial intelligence also lacks integration. It may be excellent at vision, language, or calculations, but these abilities exist in isolation and do not integrate into a unified living experience. In the human body, every system is interconnected. Emotional stress alters hormones, hormones affect immunity, immunity influences inflammation, inflammation impacts metabolism, and metabolism affects brain function. This means the body does not think, feel, digest, heal, or move separately — it does everything as one coordinated intelligent organism. We can correlate this with grief can Cadise, disturbed sleep, lowered immunity, and physical weakness, showing that intelligence in the human system is not localized but distributed and integrated.

Finally, artificial intelligence is not alive, not self-originating, not self-repairing, and not self-transcending. It does not reproduce, evolve biologically, or give rise to new intelligent life. The human body, by contrast, carries genetic memory across generations, evolves over centuries, and generates new conscious beings. It contains the instructions to build itself from a single cell, to differentiate into trillions of specialized cells, and to coordinate them into one functioning person. From a biological engineering viewpoint, this makes the human body not merely more intelligent than artificial intelligence, but categorically different — it is a living, conscious, adaptive, self-healing intelligence system, whereas artificial intelligence is a sophisticated but narrow computational tool.

In summary, artificial intelligence represents a powerful extension of human logical processing, but it is not intelligence in the full biological sense. The human body embodies intelligence as life itself — intelligence that senses, feels, repairs, protects, adapts, learns, reproduces, and gives meaning to existence. Machines can assist human intelligence, but they cannot replace, replicate, or surpass the integrated, living intelligence that operates within every human being. This makes the human body's intelligence not only superior but fundamentally irreplaceable in the natural order of life.

11.2 Origin of Intelligence

Artificial Intelligence is created by humans. It is designed, coded, trained, powered, and maintained externally. It has no independent existence. If electricity stops, it ceases instantly. If humans stop maintaining it, it degrades and fails.

Human Body Intelligence is self-originating. It begins at conception and organizes trillions of cells into a coherent, functioning organism without any external programmer. It constructs its own hardware (organs), software (neural and hormonal networks), repair systems (immune and stem cell mechanisms), and energy systems (mitochondria) automatically.

Illustration:
AI is like a robot assembled in a factory.
The human body is like a self-building, self-repairing city that designs, constructs, powers, protects, and upgrades itself continuously.

11.3 Scope of Intelligence

The scope of artificial intelligence is inherently narrow and limited to the specific functions for which it is designed. An AI system may be highly efficient at recognizing faces, translating languages, analyzing X-rays, predicting stock trends, or answering questions, but it cannot move beyond the boundaries of its training and programming. Outside its defined domain, it becomes ineffective or produces meaningless output. For example, a program trained to analyze medical scans cannot understand legal documents, human emotions, social relationships, or moral dilemmas unless separate systems are built for each task. Even then, these remain isolated abilities that do not combine into a unified understanding of life or reality.

Human intelligence, in contrast, is broad, integrated, and general in scope. A human being can think logically, feel emotionally, judge ethically, imagine creatively, remember past experiences, anticipate future outcomes, and adapt behavior accordingly — all at the same time. Humans can switch between tasks effortlessly: a person can solve a mathematical problem, comfort a crying child, plan a journey, reflect on a moral issue, and appreciate music within the same hour. This flexibility is not preprogrammed for each task; it emerges from a unified conscious intelligence that integrates perception, memory, emotion, values, and experience into meaningful understanding.

Artificial intelligence processes symbols, patterns, and probabilities, but it does not understand meaning. When an AI identifies a tumor on a scan, it is detecting statistical deviations in pixel patterns based on prior data. It does not know what cancer is, what death is, what suffering is, or what the diagnosis means for the patient's family, career, emotions, or future. The human doctor, however, understands not only the medical data but also the human context. The doctor recognizes the patient's fear, financial worries, family responsibilities, psychological resilience, cultural beliefs, and ethical preferences, and integrates all of this into how the diagnosis is communicated and how treatment is chosen.

Human intelligence is also deeply contextual and adaptive. People modify their behavior depending on who they are speaking to, where they are, what time it is, and what the social or emotional situation requires. The same words spoken to a child, a patient, a colleague, or a grieving person take on entirely different meanings and consequences. Artificial intelligence lacks this living context sensitivity. It can mimic tone or generate polite language, but it does not feel the emotional weight of a situation or grasp its human significance.

Another key difference is that human intelligence includes intuition and wisdom, which arise from accumulated experience and embodied understanding. A senior doctor may sense that something is wrong with a patient even before tests confirm it, based on subtle cues such as posture, tone of voice, skin color, or energy level. This intuitive integration of countless subtle signals is not easily reducible to data points and cannot be fully replicated by algorithms. It represents a form of intelligence that is experiential, embodied, and holistic rather than computational.

Finally, human intelligence includes ethical and moral reasoning. Humans consider what is right or wrong, fair or unfair, kind or cruel, meaningful or meaningless. They reflect on the long-term consequences of their actions for themselves, others, and society. Artificial intelligence does not possess values or responsibility; it merely executes objectives given to it. It cannot be morally accountable because it does not possess consciousness, intention, or free choice. This makes human intelligence not only broader in scope but fundamentally deeper in significance.

In simple terms, artificial intelligence is like a highly specialized tool that can perform certain tasks with great speed and accuracy, while human intelligence is a living, flexible, emotionally aware, ethically guided, and meaning-oriented system that understands life as a whole. This makes human intelligence general and universal in scope, whereas artificial intelligence remains narrow, task-bound, and fundamentally limited.

11.4 Energy Efficiency

One of the most remarkable and often overlooked differences between artificial intelligence and human body intelligence is energy efficiency. Artificial intelligence systems require enormous amounts of electrical power to perform even narrow cognitive tasks. Large data centers consume gigawatts of electricity, require constant cooling to prevent overheating, and depend on massive physical infrastructure to support servers, processors, and storage units. All of this energy is spent to simulate small fragments of what the human brain does naturally — such as recognizing images, processing language, or playing strategy games. Even then, these systems remain limited to specific tasks and cannot function without continuous external power supply and maintenance.

In contrast, the human brain operates on approximately 20 watts of power, roughly equivalent to the energy used by a dim household light bulb. With this tiny amount of energy, it performs astonishingly complex functions simultaneously. It processes visual and auditory input, controls muscle movement, regulates breathing and heart rate, manages hormonal secretion, coordinates immune responses, stores memories, generates emotions, enables learning, and supports consciousness itself — all in real time and without interruption. This level of performance per unit of energy is unmatched by any artificial system humans have ever created.

From a layman's perspective, this difference is like comparing a massive industrial factory that needs its own power station to operate a single machine, with a tiny battery-powered device that performs thousands of functions at once. A data center needs cooling plants, backup generators, technicians, and constant electricity just to keep running. The human brain needs only food, oxygen, water, and rest — and converts these simple biological fuels into electrical and chemical signals with extraordinary efficiency.

Another important aspect is that the human body not only uses energy efficiently but also produces and manages its own energy internally. Every cell contains mitochondria, which act as miniature power plants, converting nutrients into usable energy. This decentralized energy-production system allows the body to deliver energy precisely where it is needed, when it is needed, without large losses. Artificial intelligence systems, on the other hand, depend on centralized energy grids, long transmission lines, and complex cooling systems, all of which waste energy through heat loss and inefficiency.

Furthermore, biological intelligence automatically balances energy use according to demand. During sleep, energy consumption decreases and is redirected toward repair and memory consolidation. During physical activity or intense thinking, energy use increases only in the necessary regions. This dynamic load balancing allows the body to avoid waste and prevent overload. Artificial systems, however, often run at high power continuously, even when demand is low, leading to inefficiency and unnecessary energy consumption.

In simple terms, artificial intelligence is like a power-hungry machine that needs constant external fuel to perform limited tasks, while the human brain is a self-powered, self-regulating, ultra-efficient processor that runs an entire living organism on the energy equivalent of a light bulb. This makes biological intelligence not only more versatile and integrated, but also the most energy-efficient information processing system known in nature.

11.5 Self-Repair and Maintenance

A defining feature that separates artificial intelligence from human body intelligence is the capacity for continuous self-repair and autonomous maintenance. Artificial intelligence systems cannot detect and fix their own physical or logical damage. When hardware components degrade, overheat, or fail, or when software becomes corrupted, outdated, or insecure, human engineers must intervene. Servers need technicians, replacement parts, software patches, and scheduled shutdowns for maintenance. Without this external care, artificial systems gradually accumulate faults and eventually collapse.

The human body, in contrast, is a living, self-repairing system that maintains itself every moment of life. The skin continuously sheds old cells and replaces them with new ones approximately every three to four weeks, keeping the protective barrier intact. The lining of the gut, which is exposed to harsh digestive chemicals and microbes, renews itself every three to five days. Red blood cells circulate for about 120 days before being recycled and replaced, ensuring continuous oxygen delivery. Bones are not static structures but living tissues that are constantly broken down and rebuilt to maintain strength and adapt to mechanical load. At the microscopic level, DNA damage caused by normal metabolism and environmental exposure is detected and repaired millions of times each day, preventing genetic errors from accumulating.

The immune system acts as an intelligent surveillance and repair department, continuously scanning for abnormal, infected, or cancerous cells and destroying them before they become harmful. This happens silently and automatically without conscious awareness. When a person gets a cut, immune cells clean the wound, prevent infection, and initiate healing. When a virus enters the body, immune cells recognize it, eliminate it, and remember it for a faster response in the future. No artificial system has such autonomous internal defense and repair mechanisms.

From a common man's point of view, artificial intelligence is like a machine that needs a mechanic every time something goes wrong, while the human body is like a house that fixes its own cracks, replaces worn parts, cleans itself, and strengthens its walls automatically. You do not need to consciously command your wound to heal or your bones to strengthen; these processes occur naturally through built-in biological intelligence.

Another important difference is that the human body does not merely repair damage; it often improves itself through the repair process. Muscles become stronger after micro-injury from exercise, bones become denser with appropriate load, and the immune system becomes wiser after each infection. This adaptive repair is both restorative and developmental. Artificial systems, however, only return to their previous state when repaired and do not grow stronger or wiser through damage.

In summary, artificial intelligence is fragile and externally maintained, while the human body is resilient and internally maintained. The body's ability to continuously detect damage, initiate repair, prevent future harm, and even upgrade itself through experience makes biological intelligence vastly superior in self-maintenance and sustainability. This self-repair capacity is one of the core reasons why the human body remains functional for decades, while machines degrade rapidly without constant external support.

11.6 Learning vs Living

Artificial intelligence is often described as "learning," but this learning is purely mathematical and statistical in nature. AI systems adjust numerical parameters based on patterns found in large datasets, optimizing their outputs to match expected results. This process does not involve understanding, awareness, or experience. The system does not know what it is learning, why it is learning, or what the learned information means in the context of life. It simply modifies internal values to reduce error in predictions. This type of learning is mechanical and external, not experiential or meaningful.

Human learning, in contrast, is inseparable from living. Humans learn through direct sensory experience, emotional feedback, success and failure, social interaction, cultural norms, moral dilemmas, and conscious reflection. When a child touches a hot object, the pain creates a powerful memory that prevents future harm. When a student is praised, the emotional reward strengthens learning. When a person faces a moral conflict, their values and behavior evolve. These learning processes are not abstract; they are embodied in the nervous system, hormones, immune responses, muscle memory, and even facial expressions and posture.

Neuroscience shows that human learning physically reshapes the brain through neuroplasticity. New connections form between neurons, old ones are pruned, and entire networks reorganize in response to experience. Learning a musical instrument changes the motor cortex, hearing languages changes auditory processing, meditation changes emotional regulation centers, and trauma alters stress-response systems. This means learning is not merely information storage; it is a structural and biological transformation.

Human learning also integrates meaning and identity. A person does not merely learn facts; they learn who they are, what they value, whom they trust, what they fear, and what they aspire to become. A life experience can change career choices, relationships, worldview, and even physical health. Artificial intelligence cannot be transformed by experience in this way because it does not possess a self that can be changed.

In simple terms, artificial intelligence "learns" like a calculator updating formulas, while humans learn like living beings whose entire biology adapts and evolves through experience. Human learning is therefore not just computational but existential — it shapes the body, the mind, the character, and the direction of life itself.

11.7 Awareness and Consciousness

The most profound and unbridgeable difference between artificial intelligence and human intelligence is awareness and consciousness. Artificial intelligence has no inner experience. It does not know that it exists, it does not feel its own presence, and it does not experience the passage of time. It does not feel fear when threatened, joy when successful, sadness when something is lost, or love when someone is close. It does not perceive beauty, meaning, or purpose. It does not suffer, hope, or wonder. It simply processes inputs and produces outputs according to rules and probabilities, without any subjective inner life.

Human intelligence, in contrast, is built upon self-awareness. A human being knows "I exist." This simple fact allows reflection, identity, responsibility, and choice. Humans are aware of themselves as individuals, aware of others as separate beings, and aware of relationships between self and world. They recognize that time passes, that life changes, and that death is inevitable. This awareness gives rise to memory, planning, ambition, regret, gratitude, fear, hope, and meaning. A person can look at the past, imagine the future, and choose actions in the present based on values and goals. Artificial intelligence cannot do this because it has no inner point of view from which life is experienced.

Awareness also allows empathy. Humans can feel the pain of another person, rejoice in another's success, and suffer when someone they love suffers. This shared emotional reality forms the basis of ethics, compassion, society, and culture. A doctor comforts a patient, a mother comforts a child, a friend listens to grief — not because of logical necessity, but because of emotional understanding. Artificial intelligence can simulate comforting language, but it does not feel concern or care; it does not suffer when someone else suffers.

Awareness further creates responsibility and moral choice. Humans ask not only "Can I do this?" but "Should I do this?" They reflect on right and wrong, fairness and harm, and long-term consequences for themselves and others. This moral awareness arises from consciousness, not from computation. Artificial intelligence has no moral responsibility because it has no inner self to be responsible.

In simple terms, artificial intelligence is like a mirror that reflects information without seeing itself, while human intelligence is a living light that knows it is shining. This awareness of existence, of others, of time, of mortality, and of meaning places human intelligence in a category that no artificial system can enter. It is not just a higher level of intelligence, but a fundamentally different dimension of being.

Artificial intelligence does not possess ethical or moral intelligence. It does not know what is right or wrong, fair or unfair, kind or cruel. It can only follow rules, constraints, and objectives that humans design and impose upon it. If those rules are incomplete, biased, or harmful, the system will still execute them without hesitation or inner conflict. An AI system cannot feel guilt for harming someone, pride for helping someone, or responsibility for the consequences of its actions. It does not suffer when harm is caused, nor does it feel compelled to prevent it unless instructed to do so. Ethics in artificial intelligence is therefore external, imposed, and mechanical.

Human beings, in contrast, possess intrinsic ethical intelligence, commonly called conscience. This inner sense allows humans to judge actions not only by their outcomes but by their intentions, fairness, and impact on others. Even when no written rule exists, people often know instinctively when something is wrong — such as lying to a trusting friend, exploiting a vulnerable person, or harming someone for personal gain. This moral awareness arises from empathy, self-reflection, social bonds, and awareness of shared humanity. It is deeply rooted in human consciousness and emotional intelligence, not in external enforcement.

Ethical intelligence allows humans to restrain themselves even when they could benefit from wrongdoing. A doctor may refuse a profitable but unnecessary procedure because it could harm the patient. A judge may resist political pressure to give a fair verdict. A person may return a lost wallet even when no one is watching. These actions cannot be explained purely by logic or self-interest; they arise from moral values and internal accountability. Artificial intelligence cannot make such choices because it has no inner moral compass — only programmed objectives.

Ethical intelligence is also what allows societies to function. Laws are based on moral principles such as justice, fairness, and protection of the vulnerable. Medicine is guided by ethical commitments such as "do no harm," respect for patient autonomy, and compassion for suffering. Art reflects human values, ideals, and struggles. Relationships are built on trust, loyalty, honesty, and care. None of these can arise from computation alone; they arise from human moral consciousness.

In simple terms, artificial intelligence is like a tool that follows instructions without understanding their moral weight, while human intelligence includes an inner voice that asks, "Is this right?" before acting. This ethical dimension is not an optional feature; it is the foundation of civilization itself. Without conscience, intelligence becomes dangerous power. With conscience, intelligence becomes wisdom. This makes ethical and moral intelligence a uniquely human capacity that no artificial system can truly possess.

11.8 Integration Across Systems

Artificial intelligence exists as an isolated computational layer, separate from biology, emotions, immunity, hormones, metabolism, reproduction, and social relationships. It processes information in digital form and produces outputs, but it does not live within a body, does not maintain biological balance, and does not participate in the complex networks that sustain life. Its intelligence is confined to a single plane of computation, disconnected from physical survival, emotional meaning, chemical regulation, or biological continuity.

Human intelligence, in contrast, is distributed across multiple interconnected biological systems that work together as one integrated whole. The nervous system provides fast electrical intelligence, allowing perception, movement, thought, and reflexes. The endocrine system provides slower but powerful chemical intelligence, regulating growth, metabolism, reproduction, stress, and emotional states through hormones. The immune system acts as defensive intelligence, constantly scanning for threats and abnormalities and responding with precision and memory. The microbiome contributes symbiotic intelligence by influencing digestion, immunity, mood, and even brain function. Genetic and epigenetic systems provide long-term memory and adaptive programming across the lifespan and across generations.

These systems do not function independently; they continuously communicate and influence one another. Emotional stress alters hormone levels, which affect immunity, digestion, and sleep. Gut bacteria influence neurotransmitters that affect mood and cognition. Physical exercise strengthens not only muscles but also immune function, metabolic health, and mental clarity. Learning changes neural networks, which alter hormonal responses and even gene expression. This means that human intelligence is not localized in the brain alone but embodied throughout the entire organism.

From a layman's perspective, human intelligence is like an orchestra in which many instruments play together in harmony, while artificial intelligence is like a solo instrument playing one melody. The beauty and power of the orchestra come from coordination, timing, and integration across all sections. If even one section is out of tune, the entire performance is affected. Similarly, if hormonal balance, immune health, emotional well-being, or metabolic stability is disturbed, cognitive function and decision-making also suffer.

This multi-layered integration makes human intelligence adaptive, resilient, and meaningful. It allows humans to sense danger, heal injury, reproduce, bond socially, create culture, and find purpose — all as expressions of a single living intelligence. Artificial intelligence, however advanced, remains confined to computation alone. It is powerful as a tool, but limited as a form of intelligence. Human intelligence, by contrast, is not single-layered but multi-dimensional, embodied, and alive.

11.9 Superiority of Human Body Intelligence

The human body is superior because it is:

1. **Self-creating** — it builds itself from a single cell
2. **Self-organizing** — trillions of components coordinate without central command
3. **Self-repairing** — continuous regeneration prevents collapse
4. **Self-adapting** — it reshapes itself based on environment, stress, diet, and emotion
5. **Self-aware** — it knows that it exists
6. **Self-transcending** — it can reflect on itself and intentionally change itself
7. **Value-driven** — guided by meaning, purpose, and ethics, not only logic

AI can process information.
The human body **is living intelligence itself**.

11.10 Summary

Artificial intelligence is a tool created by human intelligence.
Human intelligence is a living, conscious, self-organizing biological miracle that no tool can replicate.
AI can simulate fragments of cognition.
The human body embodies intelligence.
Therefore, artificial intelligence will always remain **an extension of human intelligence**, never its replacement.

The greatest intelligence on Earth is not in silicon chips — it is in living cells.

– Dr. Rajesh Bhoir
Preventive Health Advocate

www.ingramcontent.com/pod-product-compliance
Lightning Source LLC
LaVergne TN
LVHW052258200926
848481LV00002B/399